BIOTECHNOLOGY RISK ASSESSMENT

Pergamon Titles of Related Interest

Grisham HEALTH ASPECTS OF THE DISPOSAL OF WASTE CHEMICALS
Halme MODELLING AND CONTROL OF BIOTECHNICAL PROCESSES
ICE EFFLUENT TREATMENT IN THE PROCESS INDUSTRIES
Moo-Young BIOMASS CONVERSION TECHNOLOGY:
Principles and Practice
Moo-Young COMPREHENSIVE BIOTECHNOLOGY, 4 Volumes
Moo-Young WASTE TREATMENT AND UTILIZATION
OTA COMMERCIAL BIOTECHNOLOGY
Perpich BIOTECHNOLOGY IN SOCIETY
Ricci & Rowe HEALTH & ENVIRONMENTAL RISK ASSESSMENT
Stanbury PRINCIPLES OF FERMENTATION TECHNOLOGY

Related Journals
(Sample copies available on request)

BIOTECHNOLOGY ADVANCES
THE CHEMICAL ENGINEER
CHEMICAL ENGINEERING SCIENCE
CURRENT ADVANCES IN GENETICS & MOLECULAR BIOLOGY
ENERGY
ENVIRONMENT INTERNATIONAL
INTERNATIONAL JOURNAL OF BIOCHEMISTRY
JOURNAL OF PHARMACEUTICAL & BIOMEDICAL ANALYSIS
NUCLEAR & CHEMICAL WASTE MANAGEMENT
OUTLOOK ON AGRICULTURE
TECHNOLOGY IN SOCIETY
WATER RESEARCH
WATER SCIENCE AND TECHNOLOGY

Electronic Databases

COMPREHENSIVE BIOTECHNOLOGY ABSTRACTS

BIOTECHNOLOGY RISK ASSESSMENT

Issues and Methods for Environmental Introductions

Edited by
Joseph Fiksel
Teknowledge Inc.

Vincent T. Covello
National Science Foundation

Final Report to the Office of Science and Technology Policy
Executive Office of the President
Report No. NSF/PRA 8502286

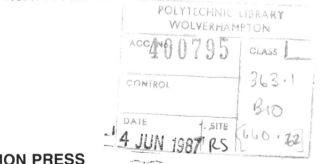
PERGAMON PRESS
New York   Oxford   Beijing   Frankfurt   São Paulo   Sydney   Tokyo   Toronto

Pergamon Press Offices:

U.S.A.	Pergamon Press, Maxwell House, Fairview Park, Elmsford, New York 10523, U.S.A.
U.K.	Pergamon Press, Headington Hill Hall, Oxford OX3 0BW, England
PEOPLE'S REPUBLIC OF CHINA	Pergamon Press, Qianmen Hotel, Beijing, People's Republic of China
FEDERAL REPUBLIC OF GERMANY	Pergamon Press, Hammerweg 6, D-6242 Kronberg, Federal Republic of Germany
BRAZIL	Pergamon Editora, Rua Eça de Queiros, 346, CEP 04011, São Paulo, Brazil
AUSTRALIA	Pergamon Press (Aust.) Pty., P.O. Box 544, Potts Point, NSW 2011, Australia
JAPAN	Pergamon Press, 8th Floor, Matsuoka Central Building, 1-7-1 Nishishinjuku, Shinjuku-ku, Tokyo 160, Japan
CANADA	Pergamon Press Canada, Suite 104, 150 Consumers Road, Willowdale, Ontario M2J 1P9, Canada

---

First printing 1986

Library of Congress Cataloging in Publication Data

Biotechnology risk assessment.

"Final report to the Office of Science and Technology Policy, Executive Office of the President."
"Report no. NSF/PRA 8502286."
Includes index.
1. Genetic engineering. 2. Microbial genetics.
3. Health risk assessment--Technique. I. Fiksel, Joseph R. II. Covello, Vincent T. III. United States. Office of Science and Technology Policy.
TP248.6.B56   1986   363.1   86-5061
ISBN 0-08-034213-2

Printed in the United States of America

Contents

List of Figures

List of Tables

Foreword

Since the publication by Professor Paul Berg and his colleagues calling for a moratorium on genetic engineering research appeared in *Nature* on July 19, 1974, a sweeping series of events have occurred. Advances in recombinant DNA research and molecular biology, and in genetic manipulation, have resulted in an impressive technology now being available for transfer of genetic material intra-, inter-, and supra-generically. Thus, in little more than ten years, a cascade of requests is flowing in to the regulatory agencies of the United States government for permission to release genetically engineered organisms to the environment for a variety of useful purposes.

Since 1974, the scientific, legal and policy issues associated with environmental applications of biotechnology have been addressed by several federal agencies. A cabinet council working group was appointed under the direction of the Office of Science and Technology Policy (OSTP), which included representatives of the U.S. Environmental Protection Agency (EPA), National Institutes of Health (NIH), U.S. Department of Agriculture (USDA), and other agencies. A proposal for a coordinated approach to the regulation of biotechnology applications was published in December 1984. Since then, a framework for federal regulation of biotechnology has been formulated that is directed at the product and not the process of recombinant DNA. The White House Biotechnology Science Coordinating Committee, chaired by Dr. David Kingsbury, Assistant Director of the National Science Foundation, has provided this framework, a refinement of the proposal published in December 1984, with the advantage that it provides a measure of regulatory certainty for industry, permitting U.S. industry to deal effectively with commercialization and to promote increased competitiveness internationally.

The issue of regulation of biotechnology is far from being closed, however, because the public will have an opportunity to comment on several proposed key definitions before the decisions become final. Public hearings will be held at the National Academy of Sciences. Additionally, three subcommittees of the House Science and Technology Committee of the U.S. Congress will hold joint hearings to review the program. As it now stands, four regulatory agencies will share responsibility for controlling organisms now covered by existing laws, including USDA, EPA, FDA and the Occupational Safety and Health Administration (OSHA). Three of the agencies, USDA, NIH and NSF, will be principally involved in overseeing research activities.

Interestingly, exceptions to federal regulation include regulating genes and deleted genes in the new framework that has been put forward. Otherwise, each agency will continue its regulatory functions, without specific reference to whether or not recombinant DNA methods were employed. Thus, the FDA will regulate human and animal drugs, medical devices and biologics, and OSHA will oversee workplace hazards. The FDA will serve as the lead agency for foods and food additives, and the USDA for food use and exclusive control over animal biologicals. The EPA will serve as the lead agency for regulating microbial pesticides released to the environment, with USDA involved if the microorganism to be released is a plant pest, animal pathogen, or a regulated article requiring a permit.

A major issue on which there is continuing debate is whether combinations of genetic material from organisms that exchange DNA by known physiological processes should be excluded from the definition of inter-generic organisms. That is, it remains to be decided whether organisms should be excluded from regulation which contain inter-generic combinations of certain specified recombinant DNA molecules which consist entirely of DNA segments from different genera that may exchange DNA by known physiological processes. Clearly, debate on this and other aspects of the regulation and control of biotechnology will continue into the future.

The focus of this book is on risk assessment of introductions of genetically engineered microorganisms to the environment. The background and motivation for study of risk assessment for such organisms, an overview of existing risk assessment approaches, available methods that can be used to assess biotechnology applications, and the suitability of the methods and their strengths and limitations are covered.

The breadth of the book is extensive in coverage of the major issues involved in risk assessment of genetically engineered organisms released to the environment. Methods for evaluation of microorganism properties, human exposure and effects analysis for genetically modified bacteria, as well as risks of human exposure to viruses as a consequence of such exposure are discussed in detail. Ecological consequence assessment, including transport and fate of bioengineered organisms in the environment, has been addressed. The value of this volume lies in the broad sweep in coverage and success in touching upon the major issues associated with release, including inter-generic genetic exchange in different ecosystems, properties contributing to environmental persistence of introduced genes and most importantly, a discussion of various risk assessment methods suitable and applicable to release of genetically engineered organisms to the environment.

Formation or creation of a genetically altered microorganism through deliberate or accidental means, deliberate release or accidental escape of these microorganisms to the environment including possible transfer of their genetic material to other microorganisms, establishment of these microorganisms within an ecosystem niche including possible colonization of humans or other biota, and subsequent occurrence of human or ecological effects arising from interaction of the organism with some host or environmental factor each require risk assessment methods. Therefore, available risk assessment methods for biotechnology applications are examined critically in this volume, with a useful model for organizing methods for risk assessment being offered.

The conclusion of the authors and of participants in the workshop is that, while methods such as ecosystem structural analysis may be useful in identifying potential risks, actual observation and testing will be essential in assuring the success and safety of environmental applications. Controlled testing and monitoring methods will be required, which include methods for detecting, identifying and enumerating specific microorganisms, methods for assessing the fate and effects of the microorganisms, and methods for assessing genetic stability of the microorganisms and the potential for genetic transfer.

Clearly, beneficiaries of attention being paid to the question of release of bioengineered organisms are the areas of microbial ecology and systematics, both disciplines having been neglected in the past mainly for not being "fashionable" or "relevant." It now appears that microbial ecology and systematics are both fashionable and relevant as well as badly needed, because of the lack of information in these disciplines to underpin decisions whether or not to release specific organisms. Fortunately, this volume will take us a significant step forward in dealing with and understanding risk and risk assessment of release of bioengineered organisms to the environment.

Rita R. Colwell
Vice President for Academic Affairs
and Professor of Microbiology
The University of Maryland

Preface

The potential applications of modern biotechnology include controlled introduction of genetically altered microorganisms into the environment for agricultural and other purposes. A number of existing scientific methods can be used to assess the risks hypothetically associated with such applications. In 1984, the National Science Foundation, at the request of the Office of Science and Technology Policy in the Executive Office of the President, initiated a study to evaluate the suitability and applicability of these scientific methods for risk assessment of environmental applications of biotechnology.

The hypothetical stages and conjectural events to be addressed in a risk assessment include:

- Formation of a genetically altered microorganism through recombinant DNA or other techniques.
- Planned release of a certain quantity of such microorganisms into the environment.
- Proliferation of the microorganism within the environment, including physical dispersal, genetic changes, or transfer of genetic material to or from other microorganisms.
- Establishment of the microorganism within an ecological niche, with or without colonization of other organisms.
- Adverse effects upon humans or the ecosystem arising from interactions of the microorganism with host or environmental factors.

Assessment of these five stages is not directly analogous to conventional risk assessment for chemical or physical agents, because microorganisms are capable of mutating, multiplying, and adapting to their environment. Microorganisms are also subject to natural barriers, competition from other species, and additional factors that tend to mitigate or prevent their proliferation and establishment. However, the capacity for proliferation and establishment is not per se problematic; in fact, it may intentionally be enhanced for beneficial purposes. Insight into these phenomena can be provided by existing methods that have been developed in molecular biology, microbial ecology, epidemiology and medicine. The major method categories addressed in this book are evaluation of microorganism properties, human exposure and effects analysis, ecosystem structural and functional analysis, environmental fate and transport analysis, ecological consequence assessment, and controlled testing and monitoring.

Chapters that describe these methods were prepared by selected experts in various disciplines. The National Science Foundation sponsored a workshop to discuss methods and to review the current state of the art of risk assessment for environmental applications of biotechnology. The principal conclusions that emerged are:

- Environmental applications of biotechnology are not a new endeavor. Microorganisms have frequently been modified in the past by methods other than recombinant DNA and have been successfully and safely introduced into the environment.
- Development of a generic approach to risk assessment for environmental applications of biotechnology is both feasible and desirable.
- The application of risk assessment methods to biotechnological products presents scientific challenges, but available methods provide a useful foundation. At the present time only a qualitative approach is feasible, since the state of the art does not permit quantitative risk assessment.
- An important requirement in the risk assessment process is detailed knowledge of the microorganism that is to be modified. One of the criteria for the selection of a candidate microorganism should be sufficiency of knowledge regarding its environmental and pathogenic characteristics.
- Microbial ecology is important to risk assessment for most microorganism introductions, and further development of this field is required. Predictive ecosystem modeling also is needed to guide and support empirical methods of risk assessment.
- Risk assessment of environmental applications of genetically engineered microorganisms should include analyses of both expected impacts and scientifically plausible, low-probability outcomes.
- Several alternative risk assessment approaches are possible, including deterministic consequence analysis with confidence bounds, qualitative screening, and probabilistic risk assessment. The choice of an appropriate risk assessment approach depends on the degree of knowledge about the microorganism and corresponding uncertainties about its characteristics under specific environmental conditions.
- At present, empirical methods such as microcosm testing are indispensable for purposes of risk assessment, but must be supplemented by predictive modeling methods.

Although risk assessment remains an inexact process, it provides a systematic means of organizing and interpreting a variety of relevant knowledge about the behavior of microorganisms in the environment.

Acknowledgments

This study was prepared by the National Science Foundation at the request of the Office of Science and Technology Policy in the Executive Office of the President. The authors gratefully acknowledge the assistance and participation of the following individuals, without whom the study could not have been completed:

Rita Colwell and John Cantlon, who served on the Steering Committee for the project.

John Cohrssen, who served as the principal coordinator on behalf of the Council on Environmental Quality and the Office of Science and Technology Policy.

David Sakura, Mildred Broome, Robert Bondaryk, Louis Anthony Cox, Patricia Deese, and John Ehrenfeld, who formed the Arthur D. Little, Inc., project team.

Sidney Draggan, who was instrumental in the conception and organization of this study.

Grant Brewen, Clint Kawanishi, Robert Rabin, Carol Scott, Sue Tolin, and Curtis Travis, who participated in an expert workshop providing many important insights contained in the book.

Joshua Menkes, who provided overall policy guidance for the project.

James Callahan, Mary Clutter, Robert Colwell, Patrick Flanagan, Robert Friedman, John Gosz, Carol Gronbeck, Frank Harris, Mark Harwell, Herman Lewis, Jonathan Plaut, Guenther Stotzky, and Peter Vitousek, who reviewed the contributed chapters.

Gloria Taylor of Arthur D. Little, Inc., who supervised preparation of the manuscript and the workshop communications.

Coordination and preparation of the contributed chapters were performed by Arthur D. Little, Inc., under Contract No. PRA-8400692 with the Division of Policy Research and Analysis, National Science Foundation, Washington, D.C.

The Suitability and Applicability of Risk Assessment Methods for Environmental Applications of Biotechnology

Joseph R. Fiksel and Vincent T. Covello

This chapter evaluates the suitability and applicability of existing methods for the assessment of conjectural risks that may be associated with environmental applications of biotechnology. The specific goals of the chapter are

- to describe and evaluate the state of the art of risk assessment for conjectural risks that may be associated with environmental releases of genetically engineered microorganisms;
- to determine the extent to which existing methods fulfill risk assessment needs, and to identify significant methodological gaps; and
- to provide a foundation and set of principles for guiding future methodological research and development.

A number of fundamental risk assessment issues are addressed:

- Does the existing risk assessment framework need to be modified to account for novel aspects of future biotechnology applications?
- What are the prospects for development of a generic risk assessment methodology for microorganisms as a complement to the case-by-case approach?
- What is the range of environmental end points that need to be considered in a comprehensive risk assessment of biotechnology applications?
- Will it be feasible in the foreseeable future to develop a capability for

risk assessment of biotechnology applications that incorporates predictive versus screening methods, probabilistic versus deterministic models, or quantitative versus qualitative results?
• Which methodology areas should be assigned highest priority in order to advance risk assessment capabilities?

The focus of the chapter is on risk assessment of planned introductions of microorganisms to the environment. Such introductions represent one of the most challenging areas for risk assessment. Many of the findings and conclusions also may be relevant to introductions of genetically modified higher organisms, such as plants or insects, as well as to inadvertent releases of microorganisms.

The chapter reviews briefly the background and motivation for this study, presents an overview of existing risk assessment approaches, discusses available methods that can be used to assess biotechnology applications, summarizes six specific categories of existing methods, and describes the results of a workshop that addressed the suitability of these methods and their strengths and limitations. Finally, we present the conclusions of the study and suggest future research priorities.

BACKGROUND

Biotechnology has been defined as the application of biological systems and organisms to technical and industrial processes [1], including such techniques as recombinant DNA, monoclonal antibodies, and cell fusion [2]. Rapid advances are taking place in the field of biotechnology, with application of these biomolecular techniques to a variety of areas such as agriculture, medicine, and chemical manufacturing [3]. New technologies, however, inevitably raise new issues [1,4,5]. One example is a recent research proposal to use genetically engineered "ice-minus" bacteria to prevent frost formation on potato and other food plants in California [6].

Scientific, legal, and policy issues related to environmental applications of biotechnology are currently being addressed by several federal agencies. For example, a Cabinet Council working group has been appointed under the direction of the Office of Science and Technology Policy (OSTP), with representatives from the United States Environmental Protection Agency (EPA), National Institutes of Health (NIH), United States Department of Agriculture (USDA), and other agencies. One product of this working group has been a proposed coordinated framework for regulation of biotechnology applications, published in December 1984 [1]. During approximately the same period, a "Points to Consider" document was drafted by a working group of the NIH Recombinant DNA Advisory Committee (RAC). This document provides guidance for submissions to the

RAC involving testing in the environment of microorganisms derived by r-DNA techniques [7].

Scientists have expressed a number of disparate views about the potential risks of releasing genetically modified microorganisms. For example, one ecologist has suggested that the outcome of introducing a new species is not predictable, since there is at present no systematic understanding of the natural factors that influence its success or failure in the environment [8]. Another ecologist has suggested that the probabilities of survival and establishment are small, but that the potential consequences may be significant [9]. A contrary view, expressed recently by an Assistant Secretary of the Department of Agriculture, suggests that "nature is resilient," and that ecological balance cannot easily be disrupted by the introduction of a genetically modified microorganism [10]. In a recent *Science* article, an industry scientist argued that the chances of adverse consequences are remote [11]. Given this diversity of views, the development of a sound risk assessment approach could be helpful in reconciling differing opinions.

The following set of Points to Consider, proposed by the RAC working group mentioned previously [7], suggests categories of information that could be included in analyzing possible risks of small-scale field tests employing modified microorganisms (see Appendix):

- Genetic considerations, including characteristics of the nonmodified parental microorganism and molecular biology of the modified organism.
- Environmental considerations (including ecological characteristics) of the nonmodified and modified microorganism, such as habitat and geographical distribution; factors affecting survival, reproduction, and dispersal; and biological or biogeochemical interactions.
- Field trial considerations, including location and conditions of the trial, anticipated effects or results, and containment and monitoring procedures.

Once this information is assembled, an analysis can be performed to evaluate whether the proposed field test might have a significant risk of undesired environmental effects.

THE RISK ASSESSMENT FRAMEWORK

In the risk assessment literature, the term "risk" generally has been defined as the potential for adverse consequences of an event or activity [12]. Risk assessment is the process of obtaining quantitative or qualitative measures of risk levels, including estimates of possible health effects and other consequences as well as the degree of uncertainty in those estimates. A recent National Science Foundation (NSF) study [13] defines risk assessment as a five-stage process:

1. *Risk identification.* Designation of the nature of the risk, including source, mechanism of action (if known), and potential adverse consequences.
2. *Risk-source characterization.* Description of the characteristics of the risk source that have a potential for creating risk (e.g., types, amounts, timing, and probabilities of release of toxic substances and energies).
3. *Exposure assessment.* Measurement or estimation of the intensity, frequency, and duration of human or environmental exposures to the risk agents that are produced by a source of risk.
4. *Dose-response assessment.* Characterization of the relationship between the dose of the risk agent received and the health and other consequences to exposed populations or to the environment.
5. *Risk estimation.* The process of integrating a risk-source characterization with an exposure and dose-response assessment to produce overall summary measures of the level of the health, safety, or environmental risk being assessed.

Table 1.1 provides a summary of available risk assessment methods; these methods are discussed in greater detail later in this chapter.

The five stages of risk assessment provide a general framework for analyzing a wide variety of risk types. The framework may be used to model both chronic risks involving ongoing exposure to risk agents, such as radiation or pollution, and acute risks associated with discrete events such as chemical spills or nuclear reactor accidents. For discrete event risks, the risk-source characterization stage often includes a "probabilistic risk assessment" to characterize the range of possible initiating events [14]. Probabilistic risk assessment involves estimating the probabilities of various adverse outcomes, which can be extremely challenging in the absence of a historical data base. When such historical data are unavailable, probability estimation is often performed using fault-tree analysis or related techniques [14]. An example of a probabilistic risk assessment is shown in Figure 1.1.

A fundamental component of a comprehensive risk assessment is a description of the range of uncertainty through the use of confidence bands or other means [15]. This uncertainty range combines both the degree of variability in the real world and the degree to which the risk model assumptions may differ from the real world. Figure 1.2 suggests how uncertainties can be propagated through the successive stages of risk assessment, resulting in a probability distributed over possible outcomes. The treatment of uncertainty in assessment of biotechnology risks is discussed later in this chapter, in the section on "Alternative Risk Assessment Approaches," which examines several alternative approaches, including both qualitative and quantitative methodologies.

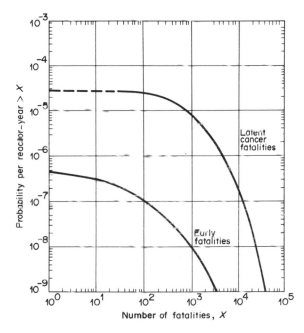

Figure 1.1. Example of risk profiles. A point (X,P) on the curve indicates that the probability is P of experiencing at least as large a consequence as X. These curves are presented as examples of the methodology only. (From Covello and Hadlock [14].)

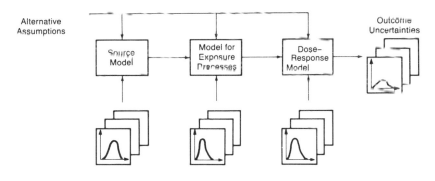

Figure 1.2. Combining models for the risk source, exposure, and dose response to obtain a risk model. (From Merkhofer and Covello [13].)

Table 1.1. Summary of Risk Assessment Methods

Risk-source characterization: Measuring the degree of hazard associated with the source of risk	Exposure assessment: Estimating the intensity, frequency, duration, etc. of human and other exposures to the risk agent	Dose-response assessment: Characterizing the relationship between the dose of the risk agent received and the health and other consequences to exposed populations	Risk estimation: Developing overall measures of the level of risk
Monitoring	Monitoring for exposure assessment	Short-term tests	Statistical analysis
Equipment monitoring	Biologic monitoring	Molecular structure analysis	Worst-case analysis
Environmental status monitoring	• food crops, livestock, fish, wild animals, indigenous vegetation, etc.	Tests on humans	Sensitivity analysis
Performance testing	Remote geologic monitoring	Animal bioassay	Confidence bounds
Accident investigation	• aerial photography, multi-spectral overhead imagery	Epidemiology	Probability distributions
Statistical methods for risk-source characterization	Media contamination (site dose monitoring)	Cohort vs. case-control Retrospective vs. prospective	Monte Carlo analysis
Statistical sampling	• air, surface water, sediment soil, groundwater	Pharmacokinetics	Event-tree analysis
Component failure analysis	Individual dose monitoring	Low-dose extrapolation models	Probability-tree analysis
Extreme value theory	• dosimeters, film badges	Animal-to-human extrapolation models	
Codified engineering methods			

Modeling methods for risk-source characterization
Engineering failure analysis
Stimulation models
• logic trees, event trees, fault trees
Analytic models
• industrial effluents, biological models for pests, containment models

Calculation of dose
Based on exposure time
Coexisting or decay substances
Material deposition in tissue
Exposure modeling
Air
• analytic models, trajectory models, transformation models
Surface water
• dissolved oxygen models, etc.
Groundwater
• absorption models
travel time models
Food chain chemical migration models
Population at risk models
Census, sensitive groups, population estimation, trip generation models, etc.

Ecological effect models

From Merkhofer and Covello [13].

AVAILABLE RISK ASSESSMENT METHODS FOR ENVIRONMENTAL INTRODUCTIONS

According to the National Science Foundation study, a risk assessment method is defined as any systematic, scientifically based procedure that can be used as a tool for risk assessment purposes [13]. A useful descriptive model for organizing methods for risk assessment of biotechnology applications was presented in a report by the Office of Technology Assessment (OTA) [16]. The model suggests a series of five events, or stages, that need to be considered in assessment. As shown in Figure 1.3, these stages correspond roughly to the three central risk assessment stages described in the previous section: risk-source characterization, exposure assessment, and dose-response assessment. The stages in OTA's model are:

1. *Formation.* The creation of a genetically altered microorganism through deliberate or accidental means.
2. *Release.* The deliberate release or accidental escape of some of these microorganisms into the environment.

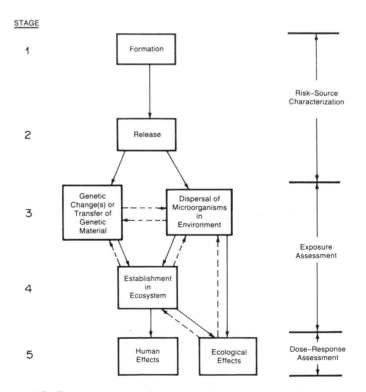

Figure 1.3. Risk assessment framework for environmental introductions.

3. *Proliferation.* The subsequent multiplication, genetic reconstruction, growth, transport, modification, and die-off of these microorganisms in the environment, including possible transfer of genetic material to other microorganisms.
4. *Establishment.* The establishment of these microorganisms within an ecosystem niche, including possible colonization of humans or other biota.
5. *Effect.* The subsequent occurrence of human or ecological effects due to interaction of the organism with some host or environmental factor.

The first two stages, formation and release, correspond to risk-source characterization. These stages can, in principle, be analyzed by quantifying the probabilities associated with various magnitudes of consequences. Estimation of probabilities and magnitudes typically is accomplished through fault-tree or event-tree analysis, or through simulation techniques, as in a recent EPA study [17].

The last stage, human and ecological effects, corresponds to dose-response assessment. This stage can, in principle, be analyzed by adapting conventional epidemiological or toxicological methods. Using such methods, a number of studies already have been conducted to assess the potential for infection and disease activation in host organisms [18]. Another extensively studied area has been the spread of antibiotic-resistant strains of bacteria in human populations [19]. Thus, existing risk assessment methods currently are being used to characterize the consequences of human exposure to biotechnology products. Ecological consequence assessment, however, is a less well-developed field and requires further research, although predictive modeling has been approached in epidemiological studies of agroecosystems. (These topics will be discussed in later sections of this chapter.)

The intermediate stages in Figure 1.3, proliferation and establishment, are difficult to analyze using existing risk assessment methods. A key difficulty is the existence of several complex "feedback loops." For example, an introduced microorganism can hypothetically transfer genetic material to microorganisms with different habitat requirements and ecological niches. Once established, microorganisms can potentially alter the environment in ways that promote further proliferation or genetic transfer, giving rise to a chain of secondary effects. Thus, for risk assessment purposes, the proliferation, establishment, and ecological effects stages cannot easily be disaggregated.

Two important areas of investigation related to proliferation and establishment are (1) environmental transport and fate of microorganisms, and (2) ecosystem interactions. Knowledge of microorganism *transport and fate* (or survival) is useful for assessing potential exposures of nontarget areas or nontarget organisms. In recent years, scientific studies of transport and fate pathways have been conducted for a variety of bacteria, algae, viruses, and other microorganisms, in conjunction with studies of wastewater treatment processes, the spread of infectious agents, pesticidal applications, and water supply protection [20]. Much of what has been learned in these studies is relevant in evaluating the transport and fate of genetically altered microorganisnms.

Potential *ecosystem interactions* between genetically modified microorganisms and other existing organisms are extremely difficult to describe or predict accurately. One approach, qualitative risk assessment, can be used to compare the propensities for survival, establishment, and genetic stability under different environmental conditions. Proliferation of the introduced or subsequently altered microorganisms might conceivably follow one of three patterns: temporary survival and eventual disappearance, establishment of one or several stable populations, or growth until limiting boundaries are reached [21]. A qualitative approach to assessing the likely pattern of ecosystem responses could circumvent the need for a full dynamic description of the events following introduction of the microorganisms.

Based upon both the OTA model and an examination of available methods, six broad categories of risk assessment methods can be identified as suitable for environmental introductions. These methods are listed in Table 1.2, along with their correspondence to the various stages of risk assessment. All six method categories are potentially useful to the risk identification stage. The last two are potentially applicable to each of the subsequent risk assessment stages. In the following section, each of these six risk assessment method categories is described and evaluated.

SUMMARIES OF SELECTED METHOD CATEGORIES

Evaluation of Microorganism Properties

A vast array of useful data exists related to microorganism persistence or persistence of genes of microorganisms used in biotechnology applications. These include data on microorganism properties that define physiological capabilities contributing to growth and persistence of the microorganism in the natural environment. Data on gene exchange and persistence are more limited but increasing. Knowing the taxonomy of organisms, particularly their genetic relationships, provides information on stable gene maintenance in the event of cross-taxon gene transfer. Environmental fate and persistence data for organisms previously released into the environment are helpful in predicting the fate of genetically engineered microorganisms.

Invasive and pathogenic properties of microorganisms for both plants and animals may enhance their potential for persistence in the environment.

Table 1.2. Categories of Methods Selected for Assessment of Environmental Introductions

	Human exposure and effects analysis	Ecosystem structural and functional analysis	Environmental fate and transport analysis	Ecological consequence assessment	Evaluation of microorganism properties	Controlled testing and monitoring
Risk identification	●	●	●	●	●	●
Risk-source characterization						
Formation					●	●
Release					●	●
Exposure assessment						
Proliferation		●	●		●	●
Establishment	●	●	●	●	●	●
Response assessment (Effect)	●	●		●	●	●

For plants, these properties include production of enzymes, toxins, or hormones that cause destruction of plant protective or structural components, inhibition of mitochondrial or specific enzyme functions, or gall formation, respectively. Virulence factors for animal pathogens include the production of a variety of factors that cause either destruction of defensive mechanisms or specific toxicity to the host.

The persistence of foreign genes released into the environment may be addressed separately from organism persistence. Presently, in vitro laboratory experiments are the principal method used for predicting potential genetic pathways in the environment, such as transfer by plasmids. Gene transfer has been demonstrated in natural environments, but more research is needed to establish the potential importance of gene transfer in the persistence and mobility of foreign genetic traits within the environment.

A fundamental concern in determining persistence is the availability of methods to detect quantitatively the presence of specific microorganisms or genes. Conventional methods to determine survivability, growth, and dispersal in a specific environment can be divided into those that (1) require growth of the microorganism on, or in, a cultivation medium or host; (2) measure biochemical activity in dilution-to-extinction media (most-probable-number methods); and (3) measure directly by microscopic observation. The first two methods require that the organism be capable of growth in available culture media. Although reliable, these methods are limited and cannot be used to describe the genetic constitution of a microorganism or to provide information about novel genes that are poorly expressed or not expressed at all. Furthermore, not all viable microorganisms can be cultured in laboratory media, including previously culturable forms that have adapted to the environment.

New methods have been and are being developed that have the potential to assess the persistence of specific genes. These nonconventional methods focus on the detection of specific DNA sequences or other DNA expression products and can be used to discriminate specific subpopulations within a complex community. Specifically, these nonconventional methods are based on (1) plasmid analysis, which is useful for plasmid epidemiology and strain detection; (2) analysis of closely linked gene cassettes, which would allow the detection of selectable genes linked to the non-selectable gene of interest; (3) protein electrophoretic analysis of gene products to discriminate among closely related phenotypes; (4) DNA/RNA probes for hybridization assays to detect and enumerate specific genotypes; and (5) restriction nuclease mapping or nucleic acid sequencing of DNA and/or RNA extracted from environmental samples.

Both conventional and nonconventional approaches to detect specific phenotypes and genotypes in the environment often depend on quantitative nucleic acid recovery and the concentration of organisms in the environmental sample. Large volume sampling of oligotrophic water containing low bacterial numbers can be performed to assure adequate nucleic acid recovery. However, extraction methodologies have yet to be developed to overcome the problem of uneven distribution of microorganisms in solid environmental samples.

In summary, the availability of preexisting information on the taxonomy, physiology, genetics, and ecology of microorganisms can contribute to an early evaluation of their environmental persistence. Furthermore, the existence of conventional methods and the development and application of new methods for detection and enumeration of specific microorganisms or genes may permit a pre- or post-evaluation of persistence.

Gaps in the available data base indicate the need to focus additional research and to integrate conventional and nonconventional approaches for determining persistence within the complex matrix of natural environments, both terrestrial and aquatic. Among the most critical data needed are information on the bioenergetics of cell and gene maintenance under environmentally realistic concentrations of available nutrients, and information on plasmid population dynamics in natural environments.

Human Exposure and Effects Analysis for Bacteria

The potential human risks of environmentally released microorganisms may be evaluated by assessing (1) the genetic and physiological characteristics of each engineered microorganism, (2) how the modified microorganism differs from the original host microorganism, and (3) any new traits that affect the ability of the engineered microorganism to persist in different ecological systems that interact with man.

Traits in microorganisms that relate directly to human disease include the ability of the microorganism to adhere to human tissues, colonize, resist antimicrobial activity of serum, produce a toxin, elicit antibodies that cross-react with host tissues, or form a capsule. The potential for transferability of "survival traits" such as these among microorganisms is important, since it would affect persistence and invasiveness. Furthermore, the potential exists for a given cloned gene to become transferable by genetic exchanges between the microorganisms being released into the environment and the microbiota normally present.

Knowledge of the ecological niche of the unmodified microorganism can be useful in predicting the ecological behavior of the genetically engineered form. Factors such as ability to utilize unusual growth substrates, tolerance of adverse physical or chemical conditions, and transportability can provide a survival advantage for a variety of microorganisms. By acquiring traits that enlarge their habitat or heighten their dominance, microorganisms may increase their potential to interact with man.

From the perspective of the human host, a number of barriers, physical and physiological, provide protection from invasion by bacteria. Outer barriers include skin, normal microflora, local antibodies, the action of cilia, and the antimicrobial action of various secretions. A second barrier that bacteria must overcome once they have entered the sterile internal environment of their target host is the immune system.

Infection depends on four major interacting factors: (1) intrinsic characteristics of the microorganism, such as invasiveness, toxin production, or resistance, which render it pathogenic; (2) number of infecting microorganisms required to overcome the host's natural defense barriers; (3) the general state of health of the individual (e.g., immunosuppression may make him or her particularly susceptible); and (4) the first and second lines of antimicrobial defense mentioned above.

One approach to evaluating the potential human health risks of an engineered microorganism is as follows: The survival and/or pathogenic traits of the microorganism can be compared with those of the unengineered microorganism from which it was derived. This should provide the pivotal prediction of pathogenicity. For most organisms known to cause infections, basic parameters such as infectious doses are available or can be obtained from animal model system studies. Assuming that the microorganism survives in the environment and contact with man occurs, laboratory studies theoretically can be done to determine whether the inserted DNA has, in any way, altered the basic nutritional and physico-chemical requirements of the microorganism. Introduced traits can be examined for their potential to affect human health. Direct studies in humans can be employed to determine the ability of organisms to colonize the gut or skin. Alternatively, in vitro tissue culture tests can help elucidate underlying cellular mechanisms and, thus, might serve as useful predictors of human infection potential or pathogenicity. Finally, the concept of "controlled eradication" of the microorganisms could be explored as a precaution, in the event that it becomes necessary.

Human Exposure and Effects Analysis for Viruses

A virus comprises nucleic acid enclosed in a protein coating that, depending upon the class of virus, may also contain a lipid envelope and/or carbohydrate residues. Viruses are intracellular parasites of many species, including man. Isolated from the intracellular environment in which they replicate, viruses may be regarded as having no independent metabolic or replicative functions. When viruses are introduced into a cell, they can mobilize cellular macromolecular synthetic mechanisms to produce more virus particles.

Evaluation of the potential for viral infection and transmission incorporates the following factors, not all of which are well understood:

- Number and severity of infections that occur in the population.
- Physiological factors that modify infection.
- Dose of virus required to cause an infection.
- Degree of horizontal transmission of the agent.
- Secretion of the agent in feces, urine, and saliva.
- Degree of viremia (dissemination of viruses by the blood).
- Propensity of the virus to remain in the population in a subclinical form.
- Mutability of the virus in nature and its effect on host resistance.
- Specific requirements of the virus for host factors that permit infection to occur.
- Host range.
- Persistence of the virus in animal and environmental reservoirs.

Naked viral nucleic acids (isolated from viruses or infected cells) can be shown under laboratory conditions to infect other cells and to transfer genetic information for integration into other cells. In most cases examined to date, however, naked nucleic acids, although having an increased host range, are significantly less infectious than the whole virus particle.

The consequences of viral infection include *lytic infection*, in which the host cell is killed and new virus particles are produced; *productive infection*, in which the host cell is not killed but new virus particles are produced and released through the cell walls; and *transformation*, in which the viral genome is integrated into the host genome, producing a permanent alteration in the host cell. Transformation may result either in a change in cell morphology or growth (e.g., neoplastic transformation, which causes a tumorous state), or in a latent infection in which pathology may not be expressed or perhaps be expressed only when the host is stressed (herpes virus) or after many years (slow viruses).

Assessment of the potential for successful viral transmission must consider a variety of interrelated factors. Survivability of viruses in the environment is influenced by their chance exposure to stresses, such as ultraviolet light, pH, and extremes of temperature and humidity. Routes of infection include respiration, ingestion, sexual transmission, fecal-oral dissemination, and direct inoculation into the skin or bloodstream by wounds or skin punctures. In each of these routes, the invading agent encounters different protective responses on the part of the host.

Host responses to the presence of viruses may include pathological effects at the subcellular level, resulting in characteristic cytopathology (abnormal structure). Classical immune response may be triggered by viral antigens which can occur at the surface of infected cells. Also, an infected host cell may become more susceptible to infection by other virus types to which it is not normally vulnerable. The physiological status of the host frequently determines the severity of a viral infection. Consequently, consideration of sensitive subpopulations is important in assessing risk.

An approach to evaluating potential human health risks of an engineered virus can be constructed in a manner analogous to that discussed in the earlier section on "Effects Analysis for Bacteria," taking into account the specific properties of viruses discussed above.

Ecological Consequence Assessment

Ecological assessment can serve at least two potential roles in a risk assessment framework. First, when the suspicion of risk is substantial, model systems can be designed to identify potential adverse effects on ecosystems before modified microorganisms are released into the environment. Second, comparative (before and after) ecological assessments can be valuable in determining whether a significant impact on ecosystem structure or function has occurred following an environmental introduction.

Ecological consequence assessments draw upon a number of approaches currently used in studies of species pathology, toxicology, and ecosystem structure and function. For instance, histological examination for tissue lesions and dose-response measurements using mortality, growth, and reproduction as end points can be important in determining effects on single species. Model multi-species systems such as microcosms can be used to evaluate the effect of perturbations on complex ecological processes such as nutrient cycling and species population dynamics. To detect differences between controls and treated field sites, ecosystem surveys can sample a variety of representative microorganisms or compare relevant biogeochemical processing rates. Effects on nonbiological components can be modeled by exposing an array of possible substrates to engineered microorganisms established in microcosm communities.

An evaluation of available test methods reveals a number of limitations associated with the current state of the art:

- Ecological systems are too complex for results from direct toxicological methods to be immediately applicable.
- Microcosm test results are often not directly comparable because of the wide diversity of testing systems currently in use, each with a narrow sphere of applicability.
- Distinguishing significant impacts from normal fluctuations in ecosystem structure requires burdensome data collection, processing, and interpretation.

- Ecosystem functional analysis alone, for example, examination of changes in biogeochemical cycles, may ignore potential shifts in population size or community composition.

Because of these limitations in empirical methods, the development of complementary predictive models is important, as will be discussed below. Nevertheless, a wealth of information can be derived from ecological assessments that monitor the effects of introducing genetically altered microorganisms on ecological structures and processes. A major challenge facing ecologists is the need to identify those end points and thresholds that are most critical and that can be addressed simply and directly. For instance, one promising approach is the development of standard methods for assessing ecologically important microorganism properties. In the interim, ecological consequence assessment can be performed through a sequence of tests. Microcosm tests of several sorts can examine potential effects on key components of ecosystems. These can be followed by more elaborate field tests that include both structural and functional measurements, with a primary focus on expected critical taxa (relationships) and processes. In addition, ecological consequence assessments can evaluate effects on nontarget processes and species, to ensure that introduced microorganisms have no unanticipated adverse consequences.

The following sections discuss in greater detail three of the most important methods that contribute to ecological consequence assessment: environmental fate and transport analysis, ecosystem structural and functional analysis, and controlled testing and monitoring.

Environmental Fate and Transport Analysis

An important aspect of risk assessment for environmental introductions of microorganisms is the evaluation of potential survival and dispersion beyond the release site. The key factors that influence possible dispersion include the size of the source population, the rate of dispersal along various environmental pathways, and the ability of the organism to survive during transport. Survival of microorganisms depends upon a number of environmental conditions, such as temperature, sunlight, moisture, nutrients, and biological interactions. Empirical studies have shown that survival times vary considerably.

The three major pathways of environmental dispersion are air, water, and vectors, including animal and technological vectors. Each is discussed below.

Viable airborne microorganisms can be transported by wind currents over long distances, and their survival may be prolonged through association with aerosols, soil, or other particles. Many of the models developed for analyzing the transport and fate of chemicals and particulates in the environment can be adapted for addressing microorganisms. These include atmospheric transport and deposition models that have been developed to describe the dispersion of pollutants from a point of release. However, further study is needed to permit reliable assessment of the transport of viable microorganisms with widely differing characteristics.

Microbial transport in surface or ground water is difficult to predict because of its dependence on complex physical mechanisms, such as attachment to particles. Computer models of runoff, surface water dispersion, and ground-water movement can be used to describe the physical transport of microorganisms, but are not presently capable of representing biochemical processes such as partitioning of microorganisms between particles and solution, or their ability to remain viable during transport.

Finally, microorganisms have been shown to be transported (1) biologically, either in the intestinal tracts, in hemolymph or salivary glands, or on the body surfaces of a variety of vertebrate and invertebrate animals; or (2) physically, on the surfaces or internal spaces of man-made materials, equipment, or vehicles, or on humans. At present few techniques exist for modeling the broad spectrum of possible mechanisms for transport by animal vectors. Transport by technological vectors is both more recognizable and more controllable.

Given the multiple pathways by which microorganisms can disperse in the environment, it appears unlikely that better than order-of-magnitude model-based prediction will be possible in the near future. One fruitful area for further research is characterization of the ability of microorganisms to survive under various conditions. Another useful research area is investigation of the nature and specificity of the interactions of microbes with their biological vectors. The results of such research would help narrow the range of known mechanisms by which microorganism might disperse and colonize new environments.

Ecosystem Structural and Functional Analysis

Understanding the overall structures and functions of ecosystems is essential in assessing the potential impacts of novel microorganisms. Structural and functional analysis provides the conceptual and mathematical tools by which such understanding can be synthesized from a more detailed knowledge of specific ecosystem compartments and the flows of energy, nutrients, and information among compartments. The structure of an ecosystem describes the interrelationships among compartments in terms of networks of these various types of flows, and its function describes the time-varying contents of the compartments. The process of ecosystem structural and functional analysis consists of four principal steps.

The first step is to aggregate the myriad of ecosystem components into compartments linked by a network of flows. Compartments may be of different types (e.g., autotrophic, abiotic, or heterotrophic) and have different importances to the ecosystem as a whole, because of either sheer physical magnitude or critical linkage (e.g., an energy or information bottleneck) with respect to other compartments in the network. Compartments can be represented at different levels of aggregation, depending on the purpose of the analysis and on technical conditions that allow meaningful aggregation of flows.

The second step in the ecosystem analysis process is to show the network of relationships that link different compartments, including flows of matter, energy, and information. Once the network has been described, structural properties such as the "connectedness" of the system, or the "vulnerability" of certain compartments to interruptions (or creations) of flows from other compartments can be established. Moreover, some ecological studies suggest that there is a relationship between network complexity, as a measure of diversity, and ecosystem stability.

After the matter/energy flows among compartments have been represented, the third step is to complete the structural description by adding the important information flows that regulate the system. Because even a small change in such control processes may, in time, become amplified into a dramatic change in system function, it is desirable to examine the impacts of introduced microorganisms at this level of analysis. Unfortunately, the structure of the control network is often poorly understood and difficult and expensive to characterize. However, even qualitative information on the sign of feedback impacts from one compartment variable to another may be valuable as a basis for analyzing the stability and the deviation-amplifying versus deviation-damping tendencies of ecological mechanisms. The behavior of the system in response to external changes can often be characterized quite satisfactorily if the general shapes of feedback functions can be specified — which in practice may be possible only if the system description is sufficiently disaggregated.

The structural analysis presented in the preceding steps is useful in the fourth step: identifying qualitatively the potential effects of introducing the microorganism into one or more compartments. To determine whether such potential effects will be realized, and to estimate their probable magnitudes, it is necessary to look beyond the structure of the ecosystem to its functional behavior, as deduced from the functional analysis of its compartments. At this point, the overall understanding of the ecosystem contributed by the structural analysis must be supported by a more detailed understanding of individual compartments and mechanisms. This deeper level of functional analysis is typically a much more data-intensive undertaking than the structural analysis.

The present state of knowledge in ecosystem analysis provides some general guidance for risk assessment of genetically engineered microorganisms. For example, the soil/sediment detritus subsystem appears especially vulnerable to introduced microorganisms, based on the structural concepts previously identified, such as low diversity and high network importance. Beyond such generalizations, however, empirical knowledge is sharply limited, making deeper analysis difficult. Current knowledge is relatively poor for information and feedback flows as compared to matter–energy flows, even though the former are perhaps the key determinants of ecosystem response to the introduction of a microorganism.

Controlled Testing and Monitoring

Successful introduction of genetically engineered microorganisms into the environment for a specific beneficial purpose will require both careful design of the introduction and a capability to evaluate and monitor its results. The latter capability involves the use of empirical methods in a systematic, stepwise fashion; such methods are indispensable for biotechnology risk assessment. While methods such as ecosystem structural analysis may be useful in identifying potential risks, actual observation and testing are essential in assuring the success and safety of an environmental application.

Controlled testing and monitoring methods can be divided into three categories: detecting, identifying, and enumerating specific microorganisms; assessing the fate and effects of the microorganisms; and assessing the genetic stability of the microorganisms and the potential for genetic transfer.

Methods for detection and enumeration of introduced microorganisms rely upon the use of various types of tracers or markers. For example, genetic markers can be used to confer a specific trait, such as antibiotic resistance, upon the microorganism. Molecular techniques, such as DNA gene probes, induction of chromogenesis, restriction nuclease mapping, or nucleic acid sequencing, can also be used for detection of introduced microorganisms.

Methods for assessing fate and effects span an array of approaches, from simple, completely contained systems (e.g., flasks, growth chambers, or greenhouses) to small-scale field trials. An increasingly important technique is the use of microcosms, which incorporate physical and biological components of an ecosystem within a closed container. There are essentially two types: naturally derived microcosms, and synthesized or standardized microcosms. The next level of testing involves introduction of the organism into controlled environments outside the laboratory. Examples include the use of greenhouses, mesocosms, or field microplots to observe the biological and ecological effects of a novel microorganism in simulated natural conditions. Further field trials in actual natural conditions are the next logical step, with appropriate means of monitoring and containment.

Methods for assessing genetic stability can be used to evaluate some of the more speculative outcomes of biotechnology applications. For example, unintended activation of certain host genes or transfer of plasmid DNA or naked DNA to other species might hypothetically result in the appearance of undesirable traits. Both of these issues can be examined through laboratory experimentation. In addition, the use of microcosms together with marker techniques will enable these issues to be investigated in a simulated complex ecosystem prior to field testing.

Although rapid improvements are being made in all of the above methods, microcosm experiments presently provide only limited insight into natural ecosystems, and the choice of microcosm components can greatly influence the results. A stepwise approach can be useful only if it is supported by meaningful correlations between observed responses in microcosms and those in mesocosm and field tests. The accumulation of a reliable data base on the ecological properties of specific microorganisms is crucial to the future assessment of the risks associated with environmental applications of biotechnology.

SUITABILITY AND APPLICABILITY
OF AVAILABLE METHODS

The risk assessment methods for environmental introductions were reviewed and discussed in an NSF-sponsored workshop attended by experts from a variety of relevant disciplines, including the authors of this book. The principal substantive conclusions of the workshop discussions are presented in this section; where no consensus was achieved, the different points of view are presented.

1. *Historical precedents for modern biotechnology.* Environmental applications of biotechnology are not a new endeavor. Microorganisms frequently have been modified in the past by methods other than recombinant DNA and have been successfully and safely introduced into the environment.

2. *Utility of risk assessment methodology.* Development of a generic approach to risk assessment for environmental applications of biotechnology is both feasible and desirable.

3. *Challenges of biotechnology risk assessment.* The application of risk

assessment methods to biotechnology products presents scientific challenges, but available methods do provide a useful foundation. At the present time only a qualitative approach is feasible, since the state of the art does not permit quantitative risk assessment.

4. *Importance of knowledge of the microorganism.* An important requirement in the risk assessment process is detailed knowledge of the microorganism that is to be modified. One of the criteria for the selection of a candidate microorganism should be sufficiency of knowledge regarding its environmental and pathogenic characteristics.

5. *Status of ecosystem analysis.* Microbial ecology is important to risk assessment for most microorganism introductions, and further development of this field is required. Predictive ecosystem modeling also is needed to guide and support empirical methods of risk assessment.

6. *Need for identification of extreme outcomes.* Risk assessment of environmental applications of genetically engineered microorganisms should include analyses of both expected impacts and scientifically plausible low-probability outcomes.

7. *Alternative risk assessment approaches.* Several alternative risk assessment approaches are possible. The choice of an appropriate risk assessment approach will depend on the degree of knowledge about the microorganism and corresponding uncertainty about its characteristics under specific environmental conditions.

8. *Empirical vs. predictive methods.* At present, empirical methods such as microcosm testing are indispensable for purposes of risk assessment, but they must be supplemented by predictive modeling methods.

The following sections elaborate on each of these points.

Historical Precedents for Modern Biotechnology

Although recombinant-DNA methods have attracted considerable attention, the theory and practice of modifying organisms are not new. Classical methods of genetic manipulation, such as hybridization, intense selection, and mutagenesis by chemicals or irradiation, have also produced modified microorganisms that were introduced into the environment with few adverse consequences. Because these techniques were less controlled and less selective than modern techniques such as recombinant-DNA, the properties of the resulting microorganisms were less predictable, and the uncertainty about potential risks would be arguably greater. However, the range of species and types of applications that are now theoretically possible exceed what was feasible with earlier techniques.

Utility of Risk Assessment Methodology

The development of a generally accepted risk assessment approach can be useful in considering proposed environmental applications of biotechnology. For example, the RAC working group's "Points to Consider Guidelines" (see Appendix) spell out the types of information that might be useful in a formal application; this information includes the characteristics of the microorganism and the experimental protocols [7]. The last section of that document requests that a risk analysis be performed based upon the above information, but it provides no guidelines for how to conduct such an analysis. The methods described in the preceding section of this chapter provide a means for such an analysis, which would interpret case-specific data in a systematic manner.

Challenges of Biotechnology Risk Assessment

Many aspects of microorganism risk assessment have precedents in previous risk assessment efforts. An important exception is the unique capability of colonies of genetically modified microorganisms to mutate, conjugate, and multiply as they proliferate, which raises the possibility of intricate interactions with existing ecosystem processes. In previous studies of energy or material releases, the system of interest has been constrained by physico-chemical laws of dissipation and decay. Even the complexities of chemical fate, food chain magnification, and metabolism can be encompassed within these constraints, and steady-state approximations are usually feasible. However, risk assessment of environmental introductions of a genetically engineered microorganism must also consider its "auto-catalytic" ability to conjugate, adapt, and multiply within its environment, thus resisting the entropic processes that govern inanimate materials. Furthermore, ecological effects from an introduction can result in additional multiplication and adaptation of the microorganism.

These auto-catalytic and feedback characteristics raise difficulties in the exposure and dose-response assessment stages of risk assessment. The concept of "exposure" is in many cases not adequate as a descriptor for environmental introduction of microorganisms, since human or ecosystem effects are unlikely to exhibit a simple exposure–response relationship. For example, infection of a specific host by an inoculation of bacteria could hypothetically have multi-species, population-wide direct and indirect impacts. Thus, the conventional separation between exposure and response appears to be an inadequate model for assessment of biotechnology risks.

Another challenging characteristic of biotechnology risk assessment is the multiplicity of human and ecological consequences that could be considered. For example, a recent workshop sponsored by the Environmental Protection Agency [22] identified several important categories of potential ecological and evolutionary impacts.

Genetic

- Rate and nature of horizontal (infectious) genetic transmission.
- Stability of the engineered genetic changes (role of movable genetic elements).

Evolutionary

- Likelihood and nature of host range shifts.
- Likelihood of unregulated propagation.
- Likelihood of changes in virulence (parasites and pathogens).

Ecological

- Effects on competitors.
- Effects on prey/hosts/symbionts.
- Effects on predators/parasites/pathogens.
- Role of introduced microorganism as vector of pathogens.
- Effects on ecosystem processes (biogeochemical effects).
- Effects on habitat.

This multiplicity of end points and associated hazard mechanisms presents a substantial challenge to existing predictive modeling methods. Thus, the development of a quantitative risk assessment approach for microorganism releases appears to be beyond the current state of the art, and a qualitative risk assessment approach such as that suggested in the next section may in the near term be more realistic.

Importance of Knowledge of the Microorganism

An important consideration in the analysis of releases of microorganisms is adequate understanding of the characteristics of the original, nonmodified, parental microorganism. By selecting microorganisms such as *Escherichia coli* that have been studied extensively, genetic researchers can better predict the behavior of the modified organism under various conditions. However, it is inevitable that microorganisms other than *Escherichia coli* will be chosen for environmental applications, because of the ability of other naturally occurring microorganisms to survive and function within the environmental medium of interest. Since data on many microorganisms are sparse or nonexistent, there is a need for the development of a well-structured data base of microorganism characteristics for selected species.

The first step in characterizing the anticipated behavior of a modified microorganism in the environment is the examination of the available data on the nonmodified, parental microorganism. In the absence of such data, the next step would be to identify the most similar microorganism for which data are available. This step raises important scientific questions about the validity of extrapolating from the characteristics of known microorganisms to closely related or slightly modified microorganisms. In this regard it would be helpful to have methods for predicting the influence of genetic modifications upon specific microorganism characteristics. This type of approach would be analogous to structure–activity relationships for organic molecules.

A preliminary list of important microorganism characteristics that bear on risk assessment is presented in Table 1.3. An important step in screening a modified microorganism for potential adverse effects is to compare it with the microorganism most similar in terms of each of the characteristics listed in Table 1.3. Uncertainty about potential adverse effects of the modified microorganism may increase if the demonstrated potential for exchange of genetic material, pathogenicity, or proliferation in foreign environments is greater than that of the nonmodified microorganism. Although this information does not confirm an increased risk, it does suggest a need to study the implications of the particular effects of an environmental introduction. Indeed, the use of a simple checklist of characteristics such as Table 1.3 may be considered a simplified form of qualitative risk assessment.

Analogy-based approaches have limited applicability when little is known about the parental microorganism, similar indigenous microorganisms, or the introduction of a known microorganism into a foreign environment. Instead, microcosm and mesocosm tests and other resource-intensive

Table 1.3. Preliminary List of Microorganism Characteristics
Important for Environmental Introductions

Exposure-related characteristics	Impact-related characteristics
Persistence in the environment	Pathogenicity for humans or biota
Host range and colonizing potential in diverse environments	Potential for dominance over indigenous organisms
Transportability of propagules	Involvement in biogeochemical cycles
Potential for transfer of genetic material	Potential for depletion of important substrates

experiments may be necessary in order to obtain adequate knowledge of the microorganism's interaction with a particular ecosystem. Again, the necessity of these tests underscores the advantages of selecting a known, indigenous microorganism for biotechnology applications in order to minimize uncertainty in the subsequent risk assessment.

Status of Ecosystem Analysis

Characterization of microorganism characteristics is only the first step in analyzing the possible adverse effects of an environmental introduction. Unless a modified microorganism is essentially identical to indigenous microorganisms, its successful establishment and proliferation are likely to perturb the local ecosystem to some degree. For example, the impact may be an indiscernible transient change in species populations, or it may be a permanent structural change in the ecosystem, such as changes in the food web. Assessing the likelihood of such impacts, even for a single ecosystem, is extremely difficult. Ecosystem dynamics is one of the most complex fields of the natural sciences, and at present predictive capabilities are embryonic at best.

Because historical records of biological introductions indicate that a small number have had visible impacts on the ecosystem [21], the question arises whether genetically modified microorganisms might have equivalent impacts. One view asserts that a general approach cannot reliably answer this question, and that scientists must proceed on a case-by-case basis, using lengthy and expensive microcosm and enclosed field experiments. An alternative view is that general principles for risk assessment based on knowledge of microorganism characteristics and ecological theory can be established and validated through a modest number of well-defined experiments. This approach would both improve the risk assessment process and provide insights into available means for mitigating risks.

A critical scientific problem inhibiting significant progress in this area is the difficulty of modeling ecosystems with reasonable accuracy. Efforts at predictive modeling require consideration of a large number of possible event sequences, including transfer of genetic material to other microorganisms, complex interaction among species, and influence of environmental changes on adaptation of the introduced microorganism or its descendants. Probabilistic descriptions of such events necessarily require large amounts of monitoring data. In the absence of such data, the results are necessarily speculative and unreliable. An extensive effort in ecosystem studies, including the theoretical and supporting laboratory work, may yield useful information on potential ecosystem-level impacts of genetically engineered microorganisms.

Need for Identification of Extreme Outcomes

An important issue in biotechnology risk assessment at the ecosystem level is investigation of remote possibilities of adverse outcomes. If one conjectures a series of improbable events, one can invariably develop an hypothesis whereby a released microorganism creates a significant ecological disruption. For example, one might speculate that a genetically engineered *Rhizobium sp.* applied to soil to enhance nitrogen fixation could become highly parasitic, resulting in reduced crop yields in the short term. A more extreme hypothesis might be stated in which the *Rhizobium sp.* outcompetes other indigenous species and permanently shifts the microbiological balance, resulting in dramatic ecological changes. This type of hypothetical risk identification process (sometimes described as "worst-case analysis") is handicapped by a lack of guidelines on the degree of improbability or ultimate consequence that should be considered.

Some limitation is necessary on the identification of low-probability events, since it is generally recognized in other risk areas, such as those involving toxic pollutants, that zero risk is unachievable [23]. As a result, many have argued for establishment of a *de minimis* risk level, that is, a probability so low that the risk in question could essentially be disregarded [24]. In the case of biotechnological applications, this concept is complicated by the auto-catalytic characteristics of microorganisms as well as by the broad potential range of outcome severity, from minor reversible impacts to severe, permanent disruptions. The greater the magnitude and the less the reversibility of an adverse effect, the lower the *de minimis* probability level of occurrence. Even if there were a sufficient understanding of ecosystem dynamics to identify various possible outcomes, it would be difficult to determine how far this process of extrapolation could proceed.

Alternative Risk Assessment Approaches

The general risk assessment framework described previously provides a useful reference point to evaluate the suitability and applicability of various methods for the analysis of biotechnology risks. The process of risk assessment can be carried out in a number of ways, depending upon the degree of uncertainty about the system being investigated and the degree of precision that is desired in the analytic results. Using these two dimensions Figure 1.4 illustrates five possible approaches: hazard description, deterministic consequence analysis, consequence analysis with confidence bounds, qualitative risk screening, and probabilistic risk assessment.

As indicated in Figure 1.4, hazard description is appropriate when uncertainty is low and quantitative precision is not required. For example, a cau-

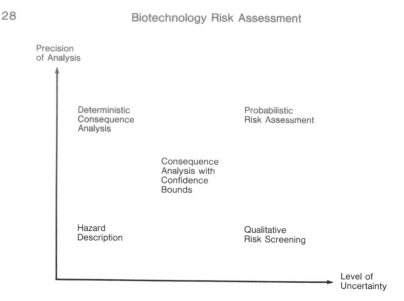

Figure 1.4. Alternative risk analysis approaches.

tionary warning about potential health effects may be adequate for
consumer product labeling, without requiring quantitative or statistical
information.

Deterministic consequence analysis is appropriate when greater quantitative precision is needed. For example, exploring the risk–benefit trade-offs
of alternative pollution control devices might require a consequence analysis to provide a quantitative basis for decision making. Where uncertainty
is low, because of extensive historical experience or a thorough understanding of the system properties, consequence analysis is usually performed in
a deterministic fashion.

Consequence analysis with confidence bounds is appropriate when uncertainties are moderate because of data gaps or complexities in the system.
In such a case, deterministic consequence analysis may be performed under
varying assumptions, thus providing confidence bounds to bracket the best
estimate of consequences [25]. Most environmental risk assessments for
chemicals are performed in this manner, although the confidence bounds
may be quite broad because of cumulative uncertainties about fate, exposure, and effects.

These three approaches are appropriate in the context of low or moderate uncertainty. However, some technological or natural systems are too
complex, and knowledge of system behavior too limited, for deterministic
analysis to capture the spectrum of possible consequences. Biotechnology
applications fall into this category only when there are no data available

on the behavior and effect of the modified microorganism in the ecosystem of interest. As pointed out earlier, the less well characterized the microorganism properties, the greater the uncertainty and the greater the requirement for empirical testing in order to assure confidence in the safety of the proposed introduction. When much uncertainty exists, as indicated in Figure 1.4, the following approaches may be used, depending on the required degree of precision.

Qualitative screening is appropriate for discriminating among different potential hazards on a relative basis. Examples of possible criteria for a screening approach based on microorganism characteristics were provided in Table 1.3. This type of approach is useful for detecting potential hazards but cannot be considered as having a predictive capability.

Probabilistic risk assessment is appropriate for obtaining quantitative a priori predictions of possible outcomes when uncertainty is high. This approach was described in the section entitled "Risk Assessment Framework."

Based on these five approaches, the following observations can be made:

• For a known indigenous microorganism with a narrowly defined genetic modification whose transport and genetic stability in the environment are relatively predictable, hazard description and deterministic consequence analysis are adequate approaches to characterizing the risks of a proposed introduction. To the extent that data gaps exist, bracketing of uncertainty will be necessary.

• For an environmental application of a nonindigenous or poorly understood, genetically modified microorganism, the uncertainty about possible outcomes will be greater, and a spectrum of scenarios must be considered. At the present time, reliable probabilistic risk analysis is not achievable because of difficulties in evaluating microorganism properties and potential ecosystem responses. Substantial progress in both molecular biology and microbial ecology is needed in order to make a truly quantitative approach feasible.

• Given the present state of the art, two options are available for dealing with moderate or greater levels of uncertainty. One is to develop qualitative screening methods for comparing anticipated risks against a benchmark or referent, and for identifying plausible worst-case or extreme scenarios. The other option is to apply exhaustive sequential empirical testing and monitoring procedures that will reduce the uncertainty to a lower level so that deterministic consequence analyses can be conducted. A logical approach is initially to use qualitative screening for detecting applications that appear to pose significant risks, and then to use more costly test methods for those applications that survive this screening.

• It may be useful to separate the biotechnology risk assessment process into two stages: an initial stage that considers the possible transient outcomes of an introduction, including the possible establishment of the microorganism in various ecological niches; and a steady-state stage that evaluates the long-term effects of the introduced microorganism, assuming the occurrence of one or more outcomes that were identified in the first stage. If the microorganism is debilitated or otherwise constrained to prevent proliferation, the second stage of analysis may not be necessary.

Empirical vs. Predictive Methods

The methods presented in the section "Selected Method Categories" can be classified into (1) mathematical models, such as dispersion models and ecosystem structural models; (2) physical simulations, for example, microcosm or mesocosm tests; and (3) real-world empirical methods, such as detection and monitoring, laboratory experiments, or field studies. As the risk assessment focus shifts from most likely outcomes to low-probability outcomes, empirically based or physical simulation methods become less useful. For example, it is unlikely that low-probability outcomes would be observed in microcosm tests or realistic field trials, although they might appear plausible based on predictive modeling studies.

The first two categories, mathematical models and physical simulations, are both modeling techniques. Although mathematical models are less costly to implement, they rely more heavily on theoretical knowledge of physical and biological mechanisms and thus require a great deal of effort to support and validate. Of the two, physical simulations appear to be the more promising predictive approach in the near future; however, a critical issue is the extent to which the results of future small-scale simulation experiments such as microcosm tests will, in fact, correlate with actual environmental outcomes.

The third category, real-world empirical methods, is an indispensable part of the risk assessment process, whether used alone or in conjunction with theoretical models. Ideally, monitoring can be used as a tool to reduce uncertainty by eventual identification and quantification of causal linkages in microorganism–ecosystem interactions. As discussed earlier, testing and monitoring of biotechnology applications (e.g., microcosm, mesocosm, or field trials) allow data gathered in one test environment to support design and justification of tests in other environments.

CONCLUSIONS AND RESEARCH ISSUES

The objective of this chapter has been to survey and evaluate the available methods for assessing the risks that may be associated with environmental introductions of genetically modified microorganisms. This chapter has focused on the description and evaluation of available scientific methods for risk assessment; no attempt has been made to assess either the existence or the range and magnitude of risks. The principal conclusions of the chapter are as follows:

- A great deal of scientific knowledge is available concerning the characteristics of nonmodified microorganisms and their interactions with ecosystems that is relevant to modified microorganisms. Knowledge from molecular biology, microbial ecology, microcosm studies, epidemiology, and other disciplines can contribute useful information to the risk assessment process.
- Risk assessment methods developed for microbiological applications in medicine and agriculture prior to recombinant DNA are equally appropriate for modern biotechnology, since the technical risk assessment issues are essentially the same.
- The development of a suitable risk assessment framework that exploits available methods is feasible. However, risk assessment approaches need to address the unique capability of genetically modified microorganisms to mutate, conjugate, and multiply.
- In addition to inference by analogy with existing microorganisms, the process of risk assessment can include a number of complementary methods: mathematical modeling, physical simulation, and real-world empirical methods (e.g., field testing and monitoring).
- The choice of an appropriate risk assessment approach will depend upon the degree of uncertainty in available knowledge, degree of desired precision, and importance assigned to the identification of low-probability outcomes.

Existing scientific knowledge and methods are adequate to perform qualitative screening of specific environmental applications, using modified microorganisms developed from microorganisms with well-defined characteristics. Further knowledge is necessary to advance risk assessment capabilities to the point where quantitative, predictive analysis can be performed for a range of modified microorganisms developed from microorganisms with poorly defined characteristics.

Promising areas of further research include:

- Development of information on properties of specific microorganisms, including habitats, persistence, dispersal, mutability, genetic transfer, pathogenicity, immunological responses, and other risk-related properties.
- Improvement in the speed, reliability, and cost effectiveness of techniques for tagging, detecting, quantifying, and assessing the vigor and persistence of microorganisms in various environments, including DNA probes, monoclonal antibodies, nucleic acid sequences, and immunofluorescent techniques.

- Development of experimental field tests that support the establishment of coherent theoretical knowledge about microbial interactions in and with ecosystems.
- Clarification of the human epidemiological significance of proliferation of drug resistance in microorganisms, and of other microbiological effects.
- Development of reliable methods, similar to the structure–activity approach for chemicals, for inferring changes in risk-related microorganism characteristics caused by specific types of genetic modifications.
- Investigation of the potential for survival of microorganisms during transport in varying states (e.g., spores, attached to particles) through foreign environments, and for subsequent establishment in new environments.
- Investigation of plasmid transfer and other ecological aspects of the fate of genetic material in the environment.
- Compilation of a data base on the characteristics of microorganisms at the ecosystem level, including inter-species interactions, population genetics, biogeochemical roles, and other relevant properties.
- Development of reliable, nonintrusive methods for containment and monitoring of field trials, including controlled eradications.
- Standardization and validation of microcosm, mesocosm, and controlled field testing protocols as predictors of the responses of selected natural ecosystems.
- Development of genetic markers that do not rely upon antibiotic resistance for detection of microorganisms in the environment.
- Development of in vitro testing strategies for assessing key microorganism properties such as pathogenicity, persistence, and invasiveness.

A suitable risk assessment framework for biotechnology applications can provide an effective instrument for integrating expertise from different scientific disciplines in a rigorous and objective manner. Although science is presently capable of tracking the consequences of environmental applications of biotechnology, pursuit of these research goals will enhance our capability to *predict* ecological outcomes for a broader range of foreseeable applications. Thus, with adequate effort, risk assessment methods for biotechnology applications can be expected to improve substantially over time. In order to minimize uncertainty about potential risks at this early stage, however, careful and purposeful selection of the microorganisms to be modified is critical.

Risk assessment is a challenging discipline, particularly in areas where historical data on potential adverse consequences are sparse. Because of limitations in both methods and data, risk assessment is an inexact process that attempts to characterize and quantify uncertainty, but never completely eliminates it. Through the systematic and rigorous application of risk assessment principles, however, existing knowledge can be organized and interpreted to provide better insight into both the possible outcomes of environmental applications of biotechnology and the available means for preventing or mitigating undesired outcomes.

REFERENCES

1. Office of Science and Technology Policy. 1984. Proposal for a coordinated framework for regulation of biotechnology: Part II. *Federal Register 49* (25):50856–50906.
2. Arthur D. Little, Inc. 1984. Federal biotechnology policy issues. Report to the National Science Foundation, Division of Policy Research and Analysis, February.
3. Office of Technology Assessment. 1983. Commercial biotechnology: An international analysis, Office of Technology Assessment, Washington, D.C.
4. Slovic, P., B. Fischoff, and S. Lichtenstein. 1980. Facts and fears: Understanding perceived risk. In R. Schwing and W. A. Albers, (Eds.), *Societal Risk Assessment: How Safe is Safe Enough?* Plenum Press, New York.
5. Gillett, J. W., S. A. Levin, M. A. Harwell, D. A. Andow, M. Alexander, and A. M. Stern. 1984. Potential impacts of environmental release of biotechnology products: Assessment, regulation, and research needs. Ecosystems Research Center, Cornell University, Ithaca, NY.
6. Milewski, E. and B. Talbot. 1983. Proposals involving field testing of recombinant DNA containing organisms. *Recombinant DNA Tech. Bull.* 6(4):141–145.
7. Department of Health and Human Services. 1985. Recombinant DNA: Notice of meeting and proposed action under guidelines for research: Part II. *Federal Register 50*(60):12456–12459.
8. Sharples, F. E. 1983. Testimony before U.S. House Committee on Science and Technology. Hearing on environmental implications of genetic engineering, June 22. Committee Print No. 26.
9. Alexander, M. 1983. Testimony before U.S. House Committee on Science and Technology. Hearing on environmental implications of genetic engineering, June 22. Committee Print No. 26.
10. Bentley, O. G. 1984. Statement before U.S. House Committee on Energy and Commerce, Subcommittee on Oversight and Investigations, December 11. U.S. Department of Agriculture, Washington, D.C.
11. Brill, W. J. 1985. Safety concerns and genetic engineering in agriculture. *Science* 227:381–384.
12. Rowe, W. D. 1977. *An Anatomy of Risk.* John Wiley and Sons, New York.
13. Merkhofer, M. and V. Covello. *Risk Assessment and Risk Assessment Methods: The State of the Art.* Washington, D.C.
14. Covello, V. and C. Hadlock, Eds. 1985. Probabilistic risk assessment: Status report and review of the probabilistic risk assessment. Document NUREG-1050, National Science Foundation, Washington, D.C.
15. Lave, L. B., Ed. 1982. *Quantitative Risk Assessment in Regulation.* Brookings Institution, Washington, D.C.
16. Office of Technology Assessment. 1981. Impacts of applied genetics: Microorganisms, plants, and animals. (OTA-BA-218). U.S. Congress, Washington, D.C.

17. Lincoln, D. R., E. S. Friber, D. Lambert, M. A. Chatigny, and M. A. Levin. 1983. Release and containment of microorganisms from applied genetics activities. Environmental Protection Agency Report, Carnegie-Mellon University, Pittsburgh, Penn.
18. Summers, M. and C. Y. Kawanishi, Eds. 1978. Viral pesticides: Present knowledge and potential effects on public and environmental health, report no. 600/9-78-026. Environmental Protection Agency, Washington, D.C.
19. Levy, S. B. 1982. Microbial resistance to antibiotics. An evolving and persistent problem. *Lancet*:83–88.
20. Berg, G., Ed. 1983. *Viral Pollution of the Environment.* CRC Press, Boca Raton, Fla.
21. Sharples, F. E. 1983. Spread of organisms with novel genotypes: Thoughts from an ecological perspective. *Recombinant DNA Tech. Bull.* 6(2):43–56.
22. Brown, J. H., R. K. Colwell, R. E. Lenski, B. R. Levin, M. Lloyd, P. J. Regal, and D. Simberloff. 1984. Report on workshop on possible ecological and evolutionary impacts of bioengineered organisms released into the environment. *Bull. Ecol. Soc. America* 65(4).
23. Ruckelshaus, W. D. 1985. Risk, science, and democracy. *Issues in Sci. Tech.* 1(3):19–38.
24. Fiksel, J. 1985. Toward a *de minimis* policy in risk regulation. *Risk Analysis* 5(4):257–259.
25. Office of Science and Technology Policy. 1985. Chemical carcinogens: A review of the science and its associated principles. Part II. *Federal Register* 50:10371–10442.

2

Methods for Evaluation of Microorganism Properties

Gary Sayler and Gary Stacey

There is a growing debate in this country over the likelihood of an environmental or health disaster as the consequence of the deliberate or accidental release of genetically engineered organisms into the environment. Respected ecologists predict an "inevitable environmental disaster" [1]. Other scientists argue, based on past experience with the release of nongenetically engineered organisms, that the chance of any such disaster is remote [2]. Yet the release of a foreign species into a new environment can have devastating consequences, as shown by the releases of the Kudzu vine, gypsy moth, Dutch elm disease, chestnut blight, and starling into the United States. Should predictions of the release of organisms or new sets of genetic traits, considered safe in their own habitat, be based upon these negative examples?

There are numerous examples of successful and beneficial releases of organisms into the environment. For example, insect release was used successfully to control troublesome weeds (*Lantana cumara*, Klamath weed) in Hawaii and California [3]. The release of the plant pathogen, *Puccinia chondrillina*, has been used successfully to control skeletonweed in Australia [3]. Presently, 13 microbial pesticide agents are approved and registered with the Environmental Protection Agency [4]. These 13 organisms are marketed in 75 different products for use in agriculture, forestry, and insect control [4]. Inoculum for leguminous plants (e.g., soybean, alfalfa, beans) has been sold in this country since the beginning of this century. The inoculum contains *Rhizobium* bacteria, which allow these plants to obtain their own nitrogen fertilizer from the air.

35

When making accurate predictions about the potential risks of the release of genetically engineered organisms, we must focus upon the previous releases of organisms into the environment and examine the literature concerning the general physiology and ecology of microorganisms. We must also define those organism properties that most contribute to risk upon release into the environment. The National Institute of Health guidelines for recombinant DNA research explicitly permit hazardous experiments to be performed only under strict conditions of confinement and with hosts that have been compromised in their ability to grow outside the laboratory [5]. Such debilitated organisms, however, would not be suitable for deliberate release into the environment, when the organism's survival is essential for achievement of a beneficial effect. The assessment of the risk of the release of any organism into the environment involves an evaluation of that organism's ability to survive, reproduce, and become established or transported into the environment. Additionally, the organism's invasive or pathogenic properties should be evaluated. A genetically engineered organism carrying foreign genes should be assessed as to the possibility of survival, establishment, reproduction, and transport of those foreign genes with or without the host organism. Persistence of the organism or trait in the environment is the key element in this assessment. If persistence occurs, then the likelihood of risk is dependent upon the organism's ability to contact a species or environment that it can harm and upon the likelihood that the organism will induce a pathogenic state. In this case, "pathogenic" refers to an organism capable of causing harm to the environment or to another living organism. A pathogenic organism must possess one or more virulence traits. To be of widespread concern, the pathogen must have the ability to be communicable from one environment or organism to another.

ORGANISM PROPERTIES CONTRIBUTING TO ENVIRONMENTAL PERSISTENCE

Microbiology has been largely a science in which cultures of single species of microorganism have been studied. As a result, we know surprising little about how microorganisms live, interact, and grow in the mixed populations found in nature. Deductions can be made, however, from the work with pure cultures. In addition, there is a growing body of information, provided by microbial ecologists, concerning microorganisms in the natural environment. A large body of information exists describing the fundamental physiology of most classes of microorganisms. Enrichment culture techniques used to isolate microorganisms from the natural environment give us information concerning the natural habitat or host of the microbes isolated [6]. The tremendous environmental and ecological complexity of the natural environment make it impossible to predict the fate or persistence of any released organism with 100% accuracy. Consequently, there is a great need for more baseline information concerning the ecology of microbes in the natural environment.

In determining the underlying risks associated with the release of genetically engineered microorganisms, both the target of risk and the critical exposure level must be identified. In this chapter, no attempt will be made to define possible biological or ecological targets or to assess the level of exposure at which risk exists. This chapter focuses on the methodology to provide critical information on the persistence of genetically engineered microorganisms or genes in the environment. Properties contributing to invasive or pathogenic risks will also be discussed. The major objective of this chapter is to identify and focus attention on those methods and concepts that contribute to an understanding of organismal or genetic persistence. Conventional and nonconventional methodologies will be discussed. In addition, information about microbial physiology, genetics, and ecology contributing to persistence of microorganisms or the measurement of persistence will be discussed.

There is a vast array of a priori knowledge of microorganisms used in biotechnology and genetic engineering. An overview of useful data relating to organism or gene persistence is given in Table 2.1. Organismal properties define physiological capabilities that could contribute to growth and persistence of the organism in the natural environment. For example, organisms possessing high affinity enzymes (low kinetic constant, Km) for the incorporation and utilization of growth substrates can persist for long periods in nutrient-poor conditions [7]. Knowledge concerning native environment, hosts, and optimal as well as suboptimal growth conditions can provide early indications of an organism's ability to persist in the environment. In addition, the taxonomic relationships, particularly the generic relationships, among nearest neighbors may provide immediate information on stable gene maintenance should gene transfer occur.

Evaluation of existing environmental fate and persistence data for organisms previously released into the environment or studied in the natural environment can be helpful in predicting the fate of novel organisms. Examples of organisms with available data bases include *E. coli, Salmonella spp., Vibrio cholerae* and *Vibrio parahaemolyticus, Caulobacter spp., Rhizobium spp.* among others. An examination of the literature indicates that fecal coliforms (FC) die quickly in the natural environment but may persist in low numbers for some time [8]. *Vibrio cholerae* has been reported to show long-term persistence in potable and brackish water [9,10]. The data suggest that *V. cholerae* in these studies was of indigenous origin and not derived from an animal host. Detection of *Salmonella spp.* in natural samples requires concentration and resuscitation treatments for efficient recovery and isolation [11,12]. The ecology of *Rhizobium spp.* has been

Table 2.1. Examples of A Priori Knowledge Useful
in Early Evaluation of Microbial Persistence

Properties	State of knowledge
Organismal	
Natural environment	Generally established
Natural host	Generally established
Alternate environment	Somewhat limited
Pathogenic host	Generally established
Growth form	Established
Specific inhibitors	Somewhat limited
Optimal growth	
substrate Km	Limited to select species
temperature	Generally established
salinity	Generally established
Growth factors	Limited to select species
Taxonomic status	Loosely established
Specific parasites	Limited to select species
Genetic	
Genotaxonomic relationships	Limited to select groups
Plasmid maintenance	Limited, but increasing
Bacteriophage sensitivity	Limited to select species
Gene transfer mechanisms	Limited to select species
Restriction/modification systems	Limited, but increasing
Plasmid incompatibility	Limited, but increasing

studied extensively (reviewed in [13]); the consensus of these studies is that introduced *Rhizobium* strains compete poorly with the indigenous microflora. Such information is useful in guiding the choice of organisms to be used in genetic engineering, and in evaluating the potential persistence of such organisms. Previous information is also important in developing methodological approaches for monitoring and determining the persistence of introduced species.

INVASIVE AND PATHOGENIC PROPERTIES OF MICROORGANISMS

The potential for specific microorganisms to be environmentally persistent can be enhanced by their ability to exist commensally or as pathogens within animal or plant hosts. A global example may be *E. coli* which might not exist in natural systems if it could be eliminated from all human and animal reservoirs. The smallpox virus has been virtually eradicated by eliminating the virus from the existing reservoirs. Large numbers of different bacterial, fungal, and viral parasites are maintained in reservoirs and released from infected hosts. Some of these organisms exist as opportunists or nonobligative pathogens, while others may represent obligative pathogens. In either case, invasive and/or pathogenic properties allow these organisms to infect plants or animals, increase in number, and be dispersed to other organisms in the environment.

Similar mechanisms of invasion and pathogenicity exist for both plant and animal pathogens. Plant pathogens must exist in or be transported to the environment of the plant. The occurrence of the organism is followed by direct contact with the plant and initiation of the invasion process. Possible mechanisms of invasion and infection are summarized in Table 2.2. The outer plant surface represents a highly resistant barrier to infection. Relatively few organisms can directly penetrate the boundary layer of the outer plant tissue. Other pathogens require a primary wound for entry. Some fungi, however, can directly penetrate the outer plant surface through physical pressure of the hyphal segments and enzymatic softening of the plant cutin covering. Cutin is a tough, waxy natural polyester. This enzymatic attack by cutin-degrading enzymes may represent the initiation of the pathogenic state since actual plant tissues are being destroyed. Once the outer surface of the plant is breached, the plant has a repertoire of additional defense mechanisms. An example of this is the hypersensitive response elicited by pathogens in some plants [14]. The pathogen is physically walled off by the plant and toxic secondary products (phytoalexins) are produced that kill the invading organism. Some plant pathogens can escape this defense because they do not elicit the hypersensitive response. Microbial

Table 2.2. Routes for Microbial Infection of Plants

Stage of invasion	Mechanism
Proximity to host	Natural or foreign microflora transport
Adhesion to host	Surface polysaccharides, pili
Penetration	
Indirect	
mechanical wounds	Abrasions
insects or other pests	Secondary penetration
Direct	
physical pressure	Fungal hyphae
enzyme attack	Cutinases, pectinases, cellulases
Infection	Enzymes
	Toxins
	Hormonal imbalance, growth regulation

Adapted from Agrios [15].

Table 2.3. Virulence Factors for Plant Pathogens

Property	Examples	Result
Enzymatic	Cutinase Cutin esterase Carboxycutin peroxidase	Destroys waxy plant covering
	Pectinase	Destroys pectin in plant cell wall
	Cellulase	Destroys cellulose, component providing strength and structured integrity of plant cell wall
	Amylase	Degradation of starch
	Proteases	Degradation of protein
Toxin	*Helminthosporium maydis* race T, HMT-toxin	Inhibits mitochondria function
	Alternia alternata f. sp. *lycospersici* AAL-toxin	Inhibits aspartate transcarbamylase
Hormoinal	*Pseudomonas syringae*	Auxin-induced gall formation
	Agrobacterium tumefaciens	Hormone-induced gall formation

pathogenicity of the plant is the result of enzymatic and toxin-induced damage as well as hormonal changes induced in the infected plant. These properties are briefly summarized in Table 2.3. Enzymatic properties of microorganisms result in the direct decomposition of structural components of the plant. Toxic properties result in alteration of physiology and enzyme function within the plant. Pathogen-produced or -induced hormonal changes effect the regulation of plant growth. All of these properties determine the disease etiology and can result in a diseased host plant that represents a reservoir contributing to the persistence of microorganisms.

Similar properties enhance the persistence and survival of animal pathogens in natural environments. The epidermal layers of the animal represent a barrier to infection by direct contact. Abrasion of the epidermal layers can contribute to the establishment of an infection. Infection of fish by the pathogen *Aeromonas salmonicida* occurs through abrasion of the epidermal layers [16]. Infection can also occur as the result of gastrointestinal ingestion as well as infection of the ova [16]. Once penetration of a potential host has occurred, a variety of factors contribute to the pathogenicity and virulence of the organism. A general summary of some of these properties is given in Table 2.4. As indicated by this table, these properties include a variety of enzymes and toxins. In addition, cellular components, such as capsular slime or surface antigen variation, may allow an

Table 2.4. Virulence Factors for Animal Pathogens

Factor	Action
Hyaluronidase	Facilitates spread of pathogens and toxic materials through host tissue
Coagulase	Causes resistance to phagocytosis
Hemolysins	Destroy red blood cells and other tissue
Lecithinase	Causes lysis of red blood cells and other tissue cells
Leucocidin	Kills leukocytes
Streptokinase	Dissolves human fibrin
Exotoxins	Cause degeneration of host cells; block essential metabolites
Endotoxin	Not clearly established
Capsules	Enable bacteria to resist phagocytosis

Adapted from Pelczar, Reid, and Chan [17].

animal pathogen to resist the cellular and immunological defense mechanisms of the host.

EXTREME ENVIRONMENTS AND PERSISTENCE OF MICROORGANISMS

The general discussion of properties contributing to persistence is directed toward natural terrestrial or aquatic environments. These are rigorous environments subject to varying conditions of low nutrient content, temperature, toxic agents, and so on. The ability of newly evolved or engineered organisms to persist in these environments is in part regulated by the availability of open niches. Open niches represent specific environmental roles to be filled in a general habitat. It is assumed that organisms released into the environment after genetic engineering were originally isolated from a natural environment where they occupied an existing niche. Existing nonmodified organisms will remain in that niche and compete with the introduced modified organisms unless new traits have been acquired that circumvent this competition. In most natural environments, it is unlikely that saturation of all available niches occurs. Novel organisms introduced into these environments may not have to compete with indigenous organisms. This hypothesis can be extended to more rigorous, extreme environments where, due to the habitat conditions, greater numbers of niches are unfilled. Such environments can include deep ocean waters and sediment (high pressure), arctic environments (low temperature), high salinity environments (e.g., the Dead Sea), high-temperature environments (hot springs, burning coal refuse), acidic environments (acid mine drainage), and environments of high-intensity ultraviolet light (alpine lakes). In such environments, organisms with unique adaptations (properties) may fill niches in which competition is minimal. Organismal properties allowing adaptation to such environments include ultraviolet protective pigments, thermally stable membrane lipids and enzymes, enzymes functional at high salt concentration or at high pressure, and modifications in cellular protein synthesis for adaptation to low temperature. Such properties allow bacterial and some fungal species to survive in harsh environments that will not sustain the vast majority of known microorganisms. Background knowledge of these microbial adaptations to extreme environments should be reviewed before releasing genetically engineered organisms into the environment. For example, microbes tolerant to high temperature are currently being studied for possible genetic modification to enhance the efficiency of selected industrial processes.

PROPERTIES CONTRIBUTING TO ENVIRONMENTAL PERSISTENCE OF INTRODUCED GENES

The persistence of foreign genes released into the environment must be addressed separately from organism persistence. The form and location of these genes within the introduced organism can affect persistence. The genetic analysis of microorganisms other than E. coli is in the beginning stages. Therefore, the data from E. coli must generally be extrapolated to other groups of microorganisms. Gene transfer between E. coli strains within the intestinal tract, the natural environment for E. coli, has been reported [18–22]. Many gene traits will be engineered into microbes using plasmids. Plasmids are extranuclear, autonomously replicated DNA elements found in many bacteria and yeast. Gene traits present on plasmids incapable of self-transmission are less likely to be transmitted [18,21,23]. Plasmids incapable of self-transmission, however, can be mobilized from one strain to another by the presence of a transmission-proficient (conjugative) plasmid [18,24]. Naturally occurring E. coli strains that contain conjugative plasmids are common [23–35]. Foreign genes inserted into chromosomal, not plasmid, DNA may be less likely to be disseminated. Mechanisms are known in E. coli whereby even chromosomally encoded genetic traits could be disseminated to unintended bacterial hosts. At present, there is little information about the transfer of genetic traits between species other than E. coli in their natural habitat.

Reanney, Roberts, and Kelly [26] have discussed possible relationships between gene exchange and interactions in natural microbial communities. Knowledge of such potential interactions can be useful in predicting the persistence of particular genetic traits in the environment. Several possible routes of intergeneric genetic exchange are shown in Figure 2.1. Presently, in vitro laboratory experiments are the major available method for predicting potential genetic exchange pathways in the environment. Marginal gene transfer has been reported in soil, animal hosts, sewage, and fresh water. All of these studies have attempted to reproduce natural environmental conditions. Many such studies, however, are flawed. For example, Graham and Istock [27] reported genetic exchange among *Bacillus* species in soil. This experiment, however, was performed at unrealistically high cell concentrations (2–4×10^8 cells/gram of soil). Additionally, cells were mixed uniformly within the soil.

Bacterial growth within soil in the natural environment is heterogeneous

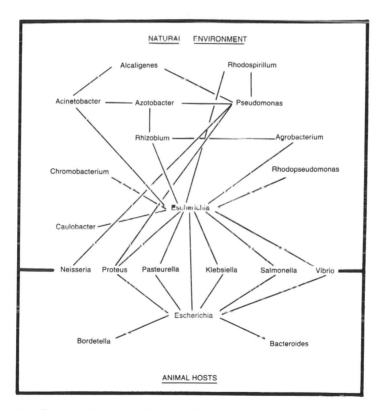

Figure 2.1. Some postulated pathways of intergeneric genetic exchange in different ecosystems. In most cases, the drawn pathways are supported by in vitro laboratory experiments. There is no evidence such transfers occur in nature. Transfers drawn are mediated by conjunction or transduction. Adapted from Reanny, Roberts, and Kelly [26].

with bacteria found within discrete microcolonies. There are a number of genetic, physiological, environmental, and ecological barriers that prohibit the free flow of genetic information among members of natural ecosystems. For example, microbes possess specific enzyme systems (nucleases) that degrade foreign DNA that enters the cell. The presence of plasmid DNA within the cell can prevent the introduction or maintenance of another closely related plasmid. In addition, experience indicates that genetic traits that are not essential (selected for) will not be maintained within the population. This is likely to be the case for many genetic traits that will be engineered into microbes. The potential importance of gene transfer in the persistence of foreign genetic traits within the environment remains an open question.

CONVENTIONAL METHODS
TO EVALUATE PERSISTENCE

A fundamental concern in determining persistence is the availability of methods to detect quantitatively the presence of specific organisms or genes in the environment. Such methods are required to determine the survivability, growth, and dispersal in an impacted environment as well as the colonization of specific habitats. Methods developed to evaluate these aspects of persistence can be divided into (1) methods that require growth of the organisms on or in a cultivation medium, (2) methods that measure biochemical activity (phenotypic expression) in dilution to extinction media (most-probable-number [MPN] approaches), or (3) direct microscopic observation. Problems and potentials of these methods have been reviewed [28,29]. These methods are limited by the requirement that the organisms be grown and by the fact that, in general, these methods lack specificity. Modifications of the cultivation media to allow for selection or screening of differential abilities may create a poor environment that further constrains quantitative extrapolation of the data. Most-probable-number approaches have been widely misused. Originally MPN tables were developed for enumeration of fecal coliforms. Some investigators use these tables without standardization to their own specific case. In other instances, conditions are standardized to one organism and then applied to mixed populations [29]. Given these limitations, however, conventional methodologies have served microbiologists well and represent the principal data base for most laboratory and field investigations. This data base represents the starting point for evaluating virtually all aspects of microbial persistence.

An available method for direct enumeration of specific bacteria in environmental samples is immunofluorescence. This method has been successfully applied to enumeration of nitrifying bacteria, *Rhizobium*, and a variety of other species (Table 2.5). In this method, an antibody specific

Table 2.5. Organisms Identified by Fluorescent Antibody
in Studies of Microbial Ecology

Organism	Type of study
Thermoplasma	Diotribution and diversity
Rhizobium japonicum	Persistence and competition
Actinomycetaceae	Identification and differentiation
Fungi	Detection and identification
Sulfolobus acidocaldarus	Growth rate, distribution, and diversity
Nitrobacter	Detection in environmental samples
E. coli	Growth rate in soil
Thiobacillus ferrooxidans	Dotoction in acid mine environment
Beijerinckia	Growth in soil
Synechococcus	Detection in lake water

Adapted from Stanley, Gage, and Schmidt [30].

to the organism of interest is tagged with a fluorescent dye. The organism in the natural sample can be detected and quantitated by the level of fluorescence. The method has received relatively little use in environmental analysis due, in part, to the need for the preparation of antibodies specific to the organisms of interest. The approach, however, does provide a potential method for in situ detection and enumeration which would be valuable in evaluating persistence. Low-density populations may require concentration to approach detection thresholds. Stanley, Gage, and Schmidt [30] have reviewed the general application of immunofluorescence and its utility. They point out that the major limitations of this method are lack of sensitivity for low population densities, lack of specificity in some applications, and the difficulty of distinguishing between viable and non-viable organisms. The specificity of immune-epifluorescent microscopy is increased by utilizing the available technology to produce monoclonal antibodies highly specific to the organism of interest.

These conventional approaches may seem limited in number; however, the number of possible modifications is extensive (Table 2.6). As long as the basic limitations of these approaches are realized, these methods are reliable. They suffer in some cases, however, from either the underestimation or overestimation of bacterial numbers and produce data with wide confidence limits. Conventional methods rely on growth or the phenotypic expression of measurable traits. These methods cannot describe an organism's genotype or provide information concerning novel genes that are poorly or not at all expressed.

The selection for antibiotic or chemical resistance by spontaneous mutation of chromosomal genes can be used to obtain organisms useful in eval-

Table 2.6. Conventional Methods for the Evaluation of Microbial Persistence

Methods	Principle	Use
Cultivation	Growth	Detection, isolation, enumeration
Enrichment	Specific carbon or energy source	Detection, isolation
Plating	Growth on solid surface	Enumeration
Selective	Selective inhibition of growth	Detection, isolation
Antibiotic resistance	Specific selection by growth	Detection, enumeration
Differential	Specific detection by activity	Detection, isolation
Most probable number	Growth or activity	Detection, enumeration
Enrichment	Growth	Enumeration
Selective	Growth	Enumeration
Differential	Activity	Enumeration
Serology	Antigen specificity	Detection, enumeration
Fluorescent antibody	Antigen specificity	Detection, enumeration
Bacteriophage sensitivity	Infectibility	Detection

Note: Limitations discussed in text.

uating persistence. Park [8] has reviewed the literature concerning the development and use of antibiotic-resistant mutants. Streptomycin-resistant mutants have been found to be particularly useful. This method, utilizing appropriate selection with complementary antibiotics, allowed assessment of the survivability of *E. coli*, *Salmonella enteritidis*, and *Vibrio spp.* in river waters [8]. Brock [31] also has discussed the relative use of antibiotic resistance markers to study the rate of growth of specific microbial populations in their native habitats. Multiple drug-resistant markers within a single strain should be used so as to prevent loss of the trait via a single mutation. Additionally, care must be taken to assess the frequency of multiple drug resistance in the environment studied. Environmental problems caused by the release of antibiotic-resistant organisms have not yet developed. Antibiotics not in medical use should be used to provide a margin of safety.

NONCONVENTIONAL METHODS
TO EVALUATE PERSISTENCE

A variety of new methods and approaches have been or are being developed that contribute to determining persistence and evaluating risks. New developments include methods for detection of specific organisms or genes as well as the use of these methods to experimentally assess microbial persistence. Nonconventional methods for detection of specific organisms or genes are summarized in Table 2.7. These methods focus on the detection of specific DNA sequences or other cellular properties. The detection of these traits can be used to discriminate specific subpopulations within a community matrix.

Among the genetic methodologies for evaluating the persistence of specific traits is plasmid epidemiology. This approach, like many others discussed, relies initially on the pure culture isolation of plasmid-bearing strains. Plasmids are isolated by any one of a number of plasmid isolation procedures and then resolved by electrophoresis through an agarose gel. For example, *Mycobacterium* cultures harboring multiple stable plasmids have been used to examine the environmental distribution and dispersal of *Mycobacterium* originating from a reservoir associated with poultry production (J. Falkinham, Virginia Polytechnic Institute, personal communication, 1984). The analysis and comparison of plasmid profiles are refined

Table 2 7 Nonconventional Methods for the Evaluation of Microbial Persistence

Methods	Principle	Use
Plasmid analysis	Plasmid gel electrophoresis, restriction enzyme analysis	Epidemiology, strain detection
Gene cassettes	Linkage of selectable trait to gene of interest	Detection of non-selectable genes
Antibiotic resistance		
Chromogenic substrates		
Protein analysis	Polyacrylamide gel electrophoresis	Discrimination of closely related phenotypes
DNA/RNA probes	DNA/RNA hybridization	Genotype detection and enumeration
Colony hybridization		
Solution hybridization		

greatly by restriction of endonuclease digestion of the plasmid DNA and electrophoresis of the fragments to yield a plasmid restriction profile or "fingerprint." Using such an approach, the spread of plasmid mediated, antibiotic-resistant *Salmonella* from infected cattle herds to human populations has been demonstrated [32].

An approach similar to the use of antibiotic-resistant marker strains to follow survival and persistence would be to use a closely linked genetic trait to follow the gene trait of interest. The idea would be to provide an easily detected gene cassette that could be placed very close to the undetectable genetic trait of interest. The presence of the undetectable genetic trait would then be followed by assaying for the closely linked gene cassette. To our knowledge, such an approach has not been used in environmental studies. Similar methodologies, however, have been widely employed in genetic studies in the laboratory. For example, the transfer of bacterial DNA to plant cells mediated by the Ti plasmid of *Agrobacterium* has been demonstrated by assaying for a linked gene-encoding gentamycin resistance [33]. In *Rhizobium*, the genetic analysis of nonselectable symbiotic traits has been performed by following transposon-encoded drug resistance closely linked to the genes of interest [34]. The use of this methodology for environmental studies should be evaluated.

Another approach that has received little use in environmental studies is the comparison of environmental isolates using protein electrophoresis. Noel and Brill [35] used sodium dodecylsulfate-polyacrylamide gel electrophoresis (SDS-PAGE) to study the population dynamics of *Rhizobium*. One-dimensional electrophoresis was found sufficient to discern differences between *Rhizobium* isolates from different plants.

The classification performed by SDS-PAGE matched that based on serology and bacteriophage sensitivity. Current technology allows several hundred isolates to be analyzed by protein electrophoresis in a single week [13]. The drawback to this method is that the bacteria must be cultured before analysis. The advantage is that the analysis does not rely on a single, potentially unstable trait but analyzes, through the electrophoretic pattern of several proteins, a fingerprint of each strain.

Methods with potentially great utility are those that detect and describe specific DNA sequences within populations and communities of organisms. Recent developments for medical diagnostic applications of DNA or RNA probe technologies may be applicable for the detection of specific genotypes in populations from environmental and other samples. The fundamental requirement for DNA probe techniques is the possession of DNA or RNA fragments that allow specific detection of the target organisms or genes. This purified DNA or RNA serves as a template for the synthesis of radioactively or chemically labeled probes. For example, single-stranded target DNA is prepared by chemical or thermal enaturation and allowed to hybridize with a single-stranded probe to form a specific duplex containing labeled DNA. This duplex can be isolated and/or detected by a variety of procedures. Currently 32_P is the most common radioactive label for DNA or RNA probes. The presence of 32_P can be directly measured by radioactive decay or by autoradiography. Radioactive sulfur (35_S) can also be used as a label for probe preparation. A new generation of chemical and immunofluorescence labels and enzyme-linked labels has also been developed with sensitivity approaching that of 32_P. These nonisotopic probes offer numerous advantages of safety, cost, detection, and shelf life. These methods are finding immediate application in medical technology.

Techniques derived from molecular genetics and molecular biology have been employed, using the original colony hybridization format of Grunstein and Hogness [36] and Hanahan and Meselson [37], to detect catabolic plasmid DNA in environmental samples [38]. Additionally, the presence of *Salmonella* [39], *V. cholerae* [40], *E. coli* [41], and *Yersinia* [42], as well as heavy-metal resistance genes [43], has been analyzed using labeled probe hybridization techniques.

Data generated by colony hybridization are essentially frequency data on the proportion of colonies capable of growth on a given medium and scored as positive targets for the probe employed. The significance of these data is limited by the specificity of the probe employed and the ability of organisms to grow on the medium of cultivation. This need for cultivation introduces the same potential problems as discussed for more conventional approaches. Probe technologies, however, can detect even one colony containing target genes in 10^6 colonies from an environmental community. Therefore, the complete loss of specific populations due to dilution can be minimized. When coupled with an appropriate selective medium, the potential exists for the resolution of specific genotypes within subpopulations in environmental samples. A hypothetical example of such an application can be developed for fecal coliforms (FC). Fecal coliforms are indicators of domestic sewage contamination and have been well studied. Methods for FC concentration via filtration and for enrichment and selective cultivation are well established. Colonies developing on membrane filters following filtration can be subjected directly to colony hybridization procedures using highly specific DNA or RNA probes. This approach could have great utility in determining whether engineered *E. coli* strains, containing specific cloned genes and accidentally released into the environment, are capable of persistence or gene transfer within FC subpopulations in the environment. This approach suffers in terms of accuracy from the requirements of growth of all FC on the enumeration medium. This requirement becomes critical when dealing with debilitated microorganisms, such as commonly used recombinant DNA *E. coli* hosts, that may require resuscitation in a nonselective medium prior to detection. It is likely that many, if not most, organisms used for genetic engineering purposes will have this sampling requirement.

Methods and approaches exist that may avoid the problems associated with growth on a cultivation medium. Among the more conventional technologies, only methods using fluorescent antibody have been used successfully to study microorganisms in situ [30]. An alternative approach could involve direct quantitative recovery of the microbial community DNA from an environmental sample. The genes of interest could then be detected and quantified using solution hybridization to a specific probe. The fundamental requirement of this approach is the availability of methods for the quantitative recovery of DNA from a highly heterogeneous community present in an environmental sample. Methods have been developed for the recovery of DNA from soil and water communities [44]. These methods require further definition as to whether the DNA extraction is quantitative and representative of the entire microbial community. Assuming that these methods can be developed for practical application, an approach can be developed using DNA:DNA reassociation kinetic analysis as described by Britten and Kohne [45]. This approach encompasses both probe hybridization and reassociation kinetics to determine the genetic complexity of an environmental sample and the existence of target DNA in that community. The approach consists of 4 components: (1) extraction of DNA from the community, (2) denaturation and time–course reassociation of the community and probe DNA, (3) separation of the double-stranded from the single-stranded DNA, and (4) quantification of bound probe. The reassociation kinetics are described by C_0t analysis, which is the concentration and time-dependent reassociation of unique DNA sequences within the total recovered DNA. The relative rate of probe reassociation can be used to determine not only the presence of specific target DNA, but also its quantitative contribution to the total community DNA. The faster the rate of probe reassociation, the more copies of the probe DNA in the environmental sample. By using a chromosomal probe to track the genotype of the original host organism and a specific probe for cloned genes of interest, it is theoretically possible to determine if the cloned genes are transferred and/or persistent in the environmental community.

Such approaches, whether the simple probe hybridization analysis or the more complex reassociation kinetic analysis, are highly dependent on quantitative DNA recovery and the concentration of organisms in the environmental sample. For oligotrophic waters containing low bacterial numbers, it is estimated that up to 1,000 liters of water would be needed to harvest enough bacteria to assure a sufficient sample size for accurate analysis. Such large-volume sampling can be performed and has the benefit of overcoming problems of uneven distribution of microorganisms in the environmental sample. The diversity and uneven quantitative distribution of microbial populations can seriously affect the resolution of C_0t analysis. A hypothetical example is given in Figure 2.2. This figure presents curves for DNA reassociation kinetics (C_0t) based on a second-order model of DNA reassociation [37]. Curve "a" represents a simple case of the DNA reassociation of a population of 10 species of equal number with no common genes. Curve "b" represents the environmental extreme of 200 species present at an equal frequency with 5 species represented at a forty-fold higher level. It should be apparent from these hypothetical examples that changes in the composition of the community are reflected by changes in the DNA reassociation kinetics. The DNA reassociation characteristics of complex communities are difficult to decipher and may provide little resolution. Major and minor alterations of specific organisms or gene frequencies, however, can be detected by tracing the reassociation rate of a specific probe and target DNA.

CONCLUSIONS

In this chapter we have not attempted to argue whether or not microorganisms released into the environment will persist or present risks. Our position is that if a release of genetically engineered organisms occurs, the availability of preexisting information on the taxonomy, physiology, genetics, and ecology of those organisms makes possible an early evaluation of their environmental persistence. Furthermore, the existence of conventional methods and the development and application of new methods for detec-

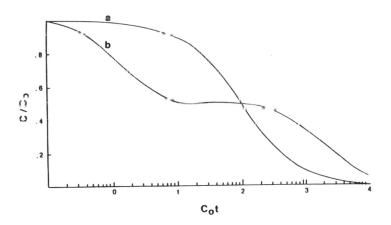

Figure 2.2. DNA reassociation kinetics for the population genomes described in the text.

tion and enumeration of specific organisms or genes makes pre- or post-evaluation of persistence possible.

What is apparent from the available data base is the need for the focusing of additional research and the integration of conventional and nonconventional approaches for determining persistence within the complex matrix of natural environments. A critical need exists for information on the bioenergetics of cell (and gene) maintenance in the presence of environmentally realistic concentrations of available nutrients. Another area lacking adequate information is plasmid population dynamics. Levin [46] presents convincing data showing that very high concentrations of nonconjugative plasmid-bearing *E. coli* are required for the persistence of that plasmid for a significant length of time in the environment. Eventually the plasmid will be lost and, even for conjugative plasmids, population dynamics will tend to inhibit maintenance of specific plasmids [46]. Knowledge of gene transfer in the environment is important for the safe and efficient engineering of organisms for environmental release.

The following conclusions are drawn from the information presented:

- In general, significant data bases exist to evaluate persistence and risk of exposure for many organisms presently employed in biotechnology.
- Where hazardous potential exists for some species, available information on specific organismal properties can direct the use of these organisms.
- Persistence in the environment is more likely to be determined by the life history or ecology of the organisms rather than by engineered traits the organisms may develop through biotechnological applications.
- Care must be taken to determine accurately the native environment of organisms to be used in biotechnology. These determinations should take into account new information about the ecology of organisms (e.g., *Vibrio cholerae*, which may have an indigenous as well as clinical environmental origin).
- Biotechnological applications of microorganisms require a significant understanding of the biochemical and genetic characteristics of the organisms. This information should be augmented by additional information on the ecology and taxonomic status of the organisms. Such analysis is necessary for accurate determination of persistence and environmental risk.
- Relatively little information exists on the persistence and transfer of genetic traits under in situ conditions. This limitation is partly overcome by knowledge of in vitro gene transfer and gene maintenance potential.
- There is a need to determine the ecological and bioenergetic parameters controlling the persistence, transfer, and reassortment of genetic information within natural community gene pools. Experience indicates that genetic traits that are not essential (i.e., selected for) may not be maintained within a population.

- Competition between indigenous and introduced organisms for available niches is likely to be a major limitation in the application and spread of released engineered organisms.
- Conventional methods for organism enumeration and determination of persistence are inherently limited by cultivation and are operative at the phenotypic level.
- The development of nonconventional methods for organism enumeration and determination of persistence contributes to understanding the maintenance and dispersal of specific DNA sequences in the environment.
- Focusing conventional and nonconventional methods on issues of genetic or organismal persistence can provide needed data for evaluating environmental risks.
- An information matrix of currently available knowledge of the physiology, genetics, and ecology of organisms, as well as experimental data on persistence, can be developed to improve the accuracy of risk assessment.

REFERENCES

1. Forcella, F. 1984. Commentary: Ecological biotechnology. *Bull. Ecol. Soc. America* 64:434–436.
2. Brill, W. J. 1985. Safety concerns regarding genetically engineered plants and microorganisms to benefit agriculture. *Science* 227:381–384.
3. Klingman, D. L. and J. R. Coulson. 1982. Guidelines for introducing foreign organisms into the U.S. for biological control of weeds. *Plant Disease* 66:1205–1209.
4. Betz, F., M. Levin, and M. Rogul. 1983. Safety aspects of genetically engineered microbial pesticides. *Recombinant DNA Tech. Bull.* 6:135–141.
5. National Institutes of Health. 1984. Guidelines for research involving recombinant DNA molecules. *Federal Register* 49:46266–46291.
6. Starr, M. P., H. Stolp, H. G. Truper, A. Balows, and H. G. Schlegel. 1981. *The Prokaryotes*, Vols. 1 and 2. Springer-Verlag, Berlin, Germany.
7. Jannasch, H. W. 1977. Growth kinetics of aquatic bacteria. In F. A. Skinner and J. M. Shewan (Eds.), *Aquatic Microbiology*. Academic Press, London, pp. 55–68.
8. Park, R. W. A. 1978. The isolation and use of streptomycin-resistant mutants for following development of bacteria in mixed cultures. In D. W. Lovelock and R. Davies (Eds.), *Techniques for the Study of Mixed Populations*. Academic Press, London, pp. 107–112.
9. Huq, A., E. B. Small, P. A. West, M. I. Huq, R. Rahman, and R. R. Colwell. 1983. Ecological relationships between *Vibrio cholerae* and planktonic crustacean copepods. *Appl. Environ. Microbiol.* 45:275–283.
10. Roberts, N. C., R. J. Siebeling, J. B. Kaper, and H. B. Bradford, Jr. 1982. Vibrios in the Louisiana gulf coast environment. *Microbial Ecol.* 8: 299–312.
11. Sayler, G. S., J. D. Nelson, Jr., A. J. Justice, and R. R. Colwell. 1976. Incidence of *Salmonellae*, *Vibrio parahaemolyticus*, and *Cl. botulinum* in an estuary. *Appl. Environ. Microbiol.* 31:723–730.
12. Kaper, J. B., G. S. Sayler, M. M. Baldani, and R. R. Colwell. 1977. Ambient temperature-primary nonselective enrichment for isolation of *Salmonella spp.* from an estuarine environment. *Appl. Environ. Microbiol.* 33:829–835.

13. Stacey, G. and W. J. Brill. 1982. Nitrogen fixation by root-inhabiting or infecting bacteria. In M. S. Mount and G. H. Lacy (Eds.), *Phytopathogenic Prokaryotes*. Academic Press, New York, pp. 225–247.

14. Sequira, L. 1978. Lectins and their role in host-pathogen specificity. *Ann. Rev. Phytopathol. 16*:453–481.

15. Agrios, G. N. 1969. *Plant Pathology*. Academic Press, New York, pp. 37–80.

16. McCarthy, D. H. 1977. Some ecological aspects of the bacterial fish pathogen *Aeromonas salmonicida*. In F. A. Skinner and J. W. Shewan (Eds.), *Aquatic Microbiology*. Academic Press, New York, pp. 299–324.

17. Pelczar, M. J., R. D. Reid, and E. C. S. Chan. 1977. *Microbiology*. McGraw-Hill, New York, p. 505.

18. Levine, M. M., J. B. Kaper, H. Lockman, R. E. Black, M. L. Clements, and S. Falkow. 1983. Recombinant DNA risk assessment studies in man: Efficacy of poorly mobilizable plasmids in biologic containment. *Recombinant DNA Tech. Bull. 6*:89–97.

19. Anderson, J. D. 1975. Factors that may prevent transfer of antibiotic resistance between gram-negative bacteria in the gut. *J. Med. Microbiol. 8*:83–88.

20. Anderson, J. D., W. A. Gillespie, and M. H. Richmond. 1973. Chemotherapy and antibiotic-resistance transfer between Enterobacteria in the human gastrointestinal tract. *J. Med. Microbiol. 6*:461–473.

21. Marshall, B., S. Schluederberg, C. Tachibana, and S. B. Levy. 1981. Survival and transfer in the gut of poorly mobilizable (pBR322) and of transferred plasmids from the same carrier *E. coli. Gene 14*:145–154.

22. Jones, R. T. and R. Curtiss. 1970. Genetic exchange between *Escherichia coli* strains in the mouse intestine. *J. Bacteriol. 103*:71–80.

23. Curtiss, R. 1978. Biological containment and cloning vector transmissibility. *J. Inf. Diseases 137*:668–675.

24. Curtiss, R. 1976. Genetic manipulation of microorganisms: potential benefits and biohazards. *Ann. Rev. Microbiol. 30*:507–533.

25. Gyles, C. L., S. Palchaudhuri, and W. K. Maas. 1977. Naturally occurring plasmid carrying genes for enterotoxin production and drug resistance. *Science 198*:198–199.

26. Reanney, D. C., W. P. Roberts, and W. J. Kelly. 1982. Genetic interactions among microbial communities. In A. T. Bull and J. H. Slater (Eds.), *Microbial Interactions and Communities*. Academic Press, London, pp. 289–322.

27. Graham, J. B. and C. A. Istock. 1978. Gene exchange and natural selection cause *Bacillus subtilis* to evolve in soil culture. *Science 204*:637–639.

28. Buck, J. D. 1979. The plate count in aquatic microbiology. In J. W. Costerton and R. R. Colwell (Eds.), *Native Aquatic Bacteria: Enumeration, Activity, and Ecology*. American Society for Testing of Materials, Philadelphia, pp. 19–28.

29. Colwell, R. R. 1979. Enumeration of specific populations by the most-probable-number (MPN) method. In J. W. Costerton and R. R. Colwell (Eds.), *Native Aquatic Bacteria: Enumeration, Activity, and Ecology*. American Society for Testing of Materials, Philadelphia, pp. 56–61.

30. Stanley, P. M., M. A. Gage, and E. L. Schmidt. 1979. Enumeration of specific populations by immunofluorescence. In J. W. Costerton and R. R. Colwell (Eds.), *Native Aquatic Bacteria: Enumeration, Activity, and Ecology*. American Society for Testing of Materials, Philadelphia, pp. 46–55.

31. Brock, T. D. 1971. Microbial growth rates in nature. *Bacteriol. Rev. 35*:39–58.

32. Holmberg, S. A., M. T. Osterholm, K. A. Singer, and M. L. Cohen. 1984.

Drug resistant Salmonella from animals fed anti-microbials. *New Engl. J. Medicine 311*:617–622.

33. Gardner, R. C. and C. M. Houck. 1984. Development of plant vectors. In T. Kosuge and E. W. Nester (Eds.), *Plant Microbe Interactions*, Vol. 1. Macmillan, New York, pp. 146–167.

34. Meade, H. M., S. R. Long, G. B. Ruvkin, S. F. Brown, and F. M. Ausubel. 1982. Physical and genetic characterization of symbiotic and auxotrophic mutants of *Rhizobium meliloti* induced by transposon Tn5 mutagenesis. *J. Bacteriol. 149*:114–122.

35. Noel, K. D. and W. J. Brill. 1980. Diversity and dynamics of indigenous *Rhizobium japonicum* populations. *Appl. Environ. Microbiol. 40*:931–938.

36. Grunstein, M. and D. S. Hogness. 1975. Colony hybridization: A method for the isolation of closed DNAs that contain a specific gene. *Proc. Natl. Acad. Sci. U.S.A. 72*:3961–3965.

37. Hanahan, D. and M. Meselson. 1980. Plasmid screening at high colony density. *Gene 10*:63–67.

38. Sayler, G. S., M. S. Shields, E. T. Tedford, A. Breen, S. W. Hooper, K. M. Sirotkin, and J. W. Davis. 1985. Application of DNA:DNA colony hybridization to the detection of catabolic genotypes in environmental samples. *Appl. Environ. Microbiol. 49*:1295–1303.

39. Fitts, R., M. Diamond, C. Hamilton, and M. Neri. 1983. DNA–DNA hybridization assay for detection of *Salmonella spp.* in foods. *Appl. Environ. Microbiol. 46*:1146–1151.

40. Kaper, J. B., S. L. Moseley, and S. Falkow. 1981. Molecular characterization of environmental and nontoxigenic strains of *Vibrio cholerae. Infect. Immun. 32*:661–667.

41. Hill, W. E., J. M. Madden, B. A. McCardell, D. B. Shah, J. A. Jagow, W. L. Payne, and B. K. Boutin. 1983. Foodborne enterotoxigenic *Escherichia coli*: Detection and enumeration by DNA colony hybridization. *Appl. Environ. Microbiol. 45*:1324–1330.

42. Hill, W. E., W. L. Payne, and C. C. G. Aulisio. 1983. Detection and enumeration of virulent *Yersina enterocolitica* in food by DNA colony hybridization. *Appl. Environ. Microbiol. 46*:636–641.

43. Barkay, T., D. L. Fouts, and B. H. Olsen. 1985. The preparation of a DNA gene probe for the detection of mercury resistance genes in gram-negative bacterial communities. *Appl. Environ. Microbiol. 49*:686–692.

44. Torsvik, V. L. 1980. Isolation of bacterial DNA from soil. *Soil Biol. Biochem. 12*:15–21.

45. Britten, R. J. and D. E. Kohne. 1968. Repeated sequences in DNA. *Science 161*:529–540.

46. Levin, B. R. and F. M. Stewart. 1980. The population biology of bacterial plasmids: A priori conditions for the existence of mobilizable nonconjugational fractions. *Genetics 94*:425–443.

3

Human Exposure and Effects Analysis for Genetically Modified Bacteria

Stuart B. Levy

Current biotechnology techniques permit the possibility of developing microorganisms for use in making a change in the environment. These organisms interact with more than one microbial species and may have direct or indirect contact with human beings. In attempting to evaluate the potential benefits versus risks of releasing changed organisms into the environment, we must be able to evaluate the consequences of such action. The literature describes the potential effects of introducing new kinds of microorganisms into already established environments. Depending on certain intrinsic (in the introduced organism) and/or extrinsic (environmental) factors, these organisms may survive, propagate, or die out. In many cases, the net result of introducing a new organism into an environment has not been predicted or considered. This chapter evaluates the potential human risks of environmentally released microorganisms by assessing the genetic and physiological characteristics of the engineered microorganism itself, how it differs from the original host organism that was altered, and how any new traits affect its ability to persist in different ecological systems that interact with man.

We now have the ability to exchange genes among different species for which there is no evidence that a natural genetic exchange can take place. Any genetic trait newly introduced into a species could potentially affect that new host, its group, its natural ecosystem, and its interaction with other organisms in its normal environment. The potential that exists for altering an entire ecosystem or for enlarging the organisms into an environment may have untoward consequences. Such was the case with the gypsy

56

moth in the United States, the mongoose in Jamaica, and the rabbit in Australia. Genetically altered species that occur naturally have demonstrated the hazards of even single gene transfer. Those creating problems for humans are generally linked to increased pathogenicity or resistance to treatment. The gene for penicillinase now found in *Neisseria sp.* and *Hemophilus sp.* is an example of natural exchange of a common gene from one group of organisms, the *Enterobacteriaceae*, into others. These new traits can greatly affect the organism's ability to exist or persist in new or altered (e.g., antibiotic-treated) environments.

The increase or decrease of one organism can affect the numbers and kinds of other members in a particular ecosystem. Such alterations could present a risk to the existence of other life forms that share or depend on that ecosystem. The results of various interactions among microorganisms in an environment could ultimately affect human beings.

FACTORS AFFECTING HUMAN EXPOSURE AND HEALTH RISKS

Intrinsic Bacterial Traits

The potential for human exposure and subsequent health risk depends on survival of the organisms. Many inherent traits of the organism itself directly or indirectly affect survival after introduction into a particular environment. The "fit" between the intrinsic traits of the organism and the extrinsic features of the environment influences the extent of survival and persistence (Table 3.1). Each organism has certain growth requirements that must be supplied by the environment. Moreover, the organism may possess survival traits that enable it to adapt and persist in the face of varied environmental factors. In regard to human risk, the organism must also be able to survive the "foreign" environment of human tissue and products. Some of these traits that relate directly to human disease are known (Table 3.2) and include the ability to adhere to human tissues, colonize, sequester trace amounts of needed iron, resist the antimicrobial activity of serum, and form a capsule. Toxin production is a pathogenic trait for which a survival feature is unknown. Many of these traits have appeared on extrachromosomal DNA elements called plasmids, which can be transferred among different bacterial species. In analyzing the importance of certain intrinsic traits (both existing and proposed) of the organism, we must know which ones can be transferred.

Under optimal laboratory conditions of excess nutrients and no competitors, most if not all extrachromosomal traits are not needed. However, in the face of environmental challenges with antibiotics, heavy metals, and

Table 3.1. Factors Affecting Human Exposure and Health Risk

Intrinsic: the organism	Extrinsic: the environment
Growth requirements	Temperature
Survival traits	Pressure
For the environment	pH
For living species	O_2 tension
For man	Humidity + H_2O content
Pathogenic traits	Electromagnetic radiation
Toxin production	Chemicals
Adherence properties	Toxic elements
Tissue tropism	Available nutrients
Intracellular growth	Ionic composition
Iron sequestration	Predators
Serum resistance	Microbial competition
Antibiotic resistance	Chance for distant spread
Genetic exchange to established members of the same and different ecosystems	

other competing strains, the ability to resist these environmental toxic elements gives a survival advantage to particular strains of bacteria. Such traits could affect the persistence of genes cloned into a resistance plasmid or a strain bearing other survival traits.

Resistance to antibiotics and heavy metals, toxin production, and many other bacterial traits can be located on movable elements called transposons, which at times reside on plasmids (transferable or nontransferable) and chromosomes. Transposons may also be picked up on bacteriophages and in this way be transferred among bacteria, although generally of more limited types. Some transposable elements, IS (insertion) elements, bear no detectable phenotype but can lead to creation of transposons. The same gene for Class A tetracycline resistance is transposable from some plasmids (e.g., pRSD1) but not from others (RPI). This feature also has been found for other genes. Thus, the potential for a cloned gene to become transposable by genetic exchanges within the organism must also be considered.

It is the genetic fluidity of the extrachromosomal transposons and plasmids that demands attention in envisioning the extent of change that could take place in the designated environment or other ecosystems when an engineered organism bearing traits on such transferable genetic vehicles is released. We highlight this factor, because it is from this environment that humans have the potential for exposure.

Table 3.2. Bacterial Traits Relating to Human Health

Characteristic	Potential human disease problem
Existing traits	
Colonization	Diarrhea
Adherence	Tissue tropism — urinary tract infec tion, endocarditis, vaginitis, etc.
Serum resistance	Septicemia
Iron sequestration	Septicemia
Antibiotic resistance	Difficult-to-treat infection
Capsule formation	Increased pathogenicity
Toxins — extracellular	Diarrhea
Degradative enzymes	Toxic by-products
Proposed engineered traits: production of	
Hormones	Physiologic effect on the host
Blood clotting factors	
Cell modulators: RNA, protein	
Viral and hormone receptors	
Genetics	
Plasmids	Genetic exchange of existing and proposed traits
Transposons	

Extrinsic Factors:
Natural Ecology of Bacteria

Bioengineered organisms are produced in the laboratory but, like other microorganisms, can find their way into the environment via the laboratory worker or movement in air, soil, and water. If they are introduced into an environment that includes agricultural products and animals, they can become part of a specific ecosystem. The ecological niche of an organism is determined by the interaction between the environment and fundamental genetic features of the organism. In order to consider the ecological range of a released engineered host-vector system, we must first know the natural ecology of the host organism itself, that is, where it can normally survive and where it is eliminated. Only then can we understand whether the bioengineered organism will persist or propagate when introduced into that environment.

Many environmental factors affect the survival of microorganisms; for example, temperature, pH, humidity, air current, and sunlight. These factors also include competition among organisms sharing the same ecosystem, as well as insects and animals that may ingest the microorganisms or transmit them to distant areas. Once delivered there, the organisms may again survive or perish. Some bacteria have learned to survive on unusual substrates, including toxic elements and inorganic salts; others resist stringent conditions of humidity and heat. These factors influence the kinds of bacteria that live in a particular environment and to what extent a bacterium can adapt to a new environment. This point is clearly evident in the evolution of bacteria that can live in a high-salt environment, but are unable to survive under physiological salt conditions. While genetically engineered traits may not totally change the natural habitat of the organism, they may enlarge the organism's area of environmental inhabitance or dominance. Subsequent to this knowledge, one can assess whether the engineered (modified) organism has an increased potential to interact with humans.

NATURAL INTERACTION OF MICROORGANISMS WITH HUMAN BEINGS

Routes of Entry: Host Defenses

What risk could newly engineered, environmentally modeled organisms have to man? To assess this potential, we must first take into account how these organisms could get into man. Humans have a natural protection against most bacterial infections: the skin. Bacteria gain entry into the sterile internal environment of human beings through abrasions and cuts in the skin. A similar kind of barrier exists throughout the intestinal tract and mucous membranes. Bacteria normally reside on skin, in the oropharynx and intestinal tract, and on other body areas exposed to the atmosphere. These naturally occurring bacteria have intrinsic traits that aid in their ability to colonize, and to protect against colonization by invading potential pathogens. Natural physiologic defenses of cellular impenetrability, local antibodies, the action of cilia, and the antimicrobial action of various secretions also protect against entry of pathogens into the body.

Having penetrated this outer, initial barrier, invading bacteria face an internal second line of defense. Circulating macrophages, monocytes, and granulocytes engulf bacteria, usually identified by serum proteins called opsonins that coat the bacteria, rendering them susceptible to granulocytic ingestion and inactivation. These cellular responses combined with the serum complement-activated lytic system and the production of antibodies, generally are a successful defense against organisms that enter the body. Factors affecting this defense are the number of organisms that enter and the state of health of the individual. The greater the number of microorganisms, the better the chance of infection.

The General State of the Individual

Individuals suffering from debilitating disease, including those being treated with chemotherapeutic agents, are at higher risk of entry and colonization by bacterial strains involved in opportunistic infections. In a study of hospitalized patients, those with more severe diseases carried increased numbers of gram-negative bacteria, including potential pathogens, in their oropharynx [10]. The results suggest an impairment in natural pharyngeal antimicrobial activities. Some evidence for decreased proteolytic activity has been presented [36]. Loss of stomach acid can also lead to colonization of the upper gastrointestinal tract. The number of organisms in the dose is critical to infection (Table 3.3). In compromised and immunocompromised hosts, a lower dose of organisms will cause an infection. Patients with cancers and leukemias, even without chemotherapy, are at increased risk of infection because of lowered natural defense mechanisms. As therapy for these diseases occurs more frequently on an outpatient basis, the number of individuals at risk in the population will increase.

Human infection thus depends on four major interacting factors: (1) the intrinsic traits, including pathogenicity, of the organisms; (2) the number

Table 3.3. Infectious Dose (25–50% of Human Volunteers)

Disease or agent	Route	Dose[a]
Bacteria		
Tularaemia	Inhalation	10
Shigella flexneri	Ingestion	180
Anthrax	Inhalation	1,300
Typhoid fever	Ingestion	10^5
Cholera	Ingestion	10^{8}[b]
Escherichia coli	Ingestion	10^{8}[c]
Parasites		
Malaria	Intravenous	10
Syphilis	Intradermal	57
Rickettsia		
Scrub typhus	Intradermal	3[d]
Q fever	Inhalation	10

From Collins [6], with permission.

[a]Number of organisms.

[b]Can be 10^3 (M. Levine, personal communication 1984).

[c]Can be 10^6 (M. Levine, personal communication 1984).

[d]Mouse ID.

of invasive organisms; (3) the general state of the individual; and (4) the first and second lines of host antimicrobial defense.

APPROACH TO RISK ASSESSMENT OF BIOENGINEERED ORGANISMS

Evaluation of the Host Microorganism

There are two genetic components to the engineered organism: its chromosome and its extrachromosomal elements. A reasonable approach to evaluating the potential health risks of engineered organisms produced in the laboratory is to know first whether the intrinsic survival and/or pathogenic traits characteristic of the unengineered host organism have been altered. Risk assessment of the engineered organisms should begin with known, testable pathogenic traits. These should be evaluated for changes based on previous monitoring and testing, in vitro and in vivo, that form the basis for categorizing the potential pathogenicity of the host organism.

Data on the infectious dose for most organisms presently under consideration have been published and are available. Comparisons are described in terms of the 50% lethal dose (LD50) or infectious dose for 25–50% of individuals (Table 3.3) [6]. Data for most organisms known to be pathogens or causing opportunistic infections are available. If not, data similar to those already provided for other organisms can be generated for any unknown ones.

An indirect measure of infection potential has come from an evaluation of various organisms' relative frequency in causing laboratory-acquired infections (Table 3.4) [6,23,24]. Eight of the top ten causes of laboratory-associated infections are microorganisms: four bacterial infections — brucellosis (1), typhoid fever (4), tularaemia (5), tuberculosis (6); one rickettsia (Q fever, 2), one chlamydial (psittacosis, 9), and two fungal infections (dermatomycoses, 7; and coccidioidomycosis, 10) (Table 3.5) [6]. On these bases, the Centers for Disease Control (CDC), the Department of Health, Education and Welfare, and other health agencies have compiled a listing of organisms with potential risk to human health (Table 3.6) [7]. These lists should be consulted in attempting to predict initially a potential risk of an organism being used as an engineered host. In general, knowing how the organism is related to other better-known organisms in its species, genera, or ecosystem will provide important defining biological features.

Some characteristics of introduced traits that could affect human health adversely are listed in Table 3.7. These potential secondary effects of genes cloned into the organism could result from altered structure (cell membrane) or production of extracellular molecules (e.g., hormones).

Table 3.4. Known Laboratory-Acquired Infections, 1930–1974

Disease or agent	No. of cases	No. of deaths
Bacterial infections		
Brucellosis	423	5
Typhoid	256	20
Tularaemia	225	2
Tuberculosis	176	4
Streptococcus	78	4
Leptospirosis	67	10
Shigellosis	58	0
Salmonellosis	48	0
Relapsing fever	45	2
Anthrax	45	5
Erysipeloid	43	0
Diphtheria	33	0
Staphylococcus	29	1
Rate-bite fever	21	0
Glanders	20	7
Syphilis	15	0
Cholera	12	4
Plague	10	4
Neisseria meningitidis	8	1
Pseudomonas pseudomallei	8	0
Clostridium	6	0
Tetanus toxin	5	0
Mixed infection	5	0
Miscellaneous bacteria	33	0
Total	1,669	69
Rickettsial infections		
Q fever	278	1
Murine typhus	68	0
Rocky Mt. spotted fever	63	11
Typhus (type not indicated)	57	0
Epidemic typhus	56	3
Scrub typhus	35	8
Trench fever	10	0
Rickettsialpox	5	0
African tick bite fever	1	0
Total	573	23
Fungal infections		
Dermatomycosis	161	0
Coccidioidomycosis	93	2
Histoplasmosis	71	1
Sporotrichosis	12	0
Blastomycosis	11	2
Other fungi	5	0
Total	353	5

continued

Table 3.4. (Continued)

Disease or agent	No. of cases	No. of deaths
Chlamydial infections		
Psittacosis	116	10
Lymphogranuloma venereum	7	0
Trachoma	5	0
Total	128	10
Parasitic infections		
Toxoplasmosis	28	1
Amoebiasis	23	0
Malaria	18	0
Trypanosomiasis	17	0
Ascariasis	8	0
Coccidiosis	5	0
Leishmaniasis	4	1
Other parasites	12	0
Total	115	2
Agent not specified	34	1
Grand total	3,921	164

From Collins [6], with permission.

Another consideration should include the concept of "controlled removal." If the need occurs, can the organisms be eliminated easily? If an antibiotic resistance gene were introduced, which specified resistance to the only antibiotic left to treat this particular organism, such action would alter the potential risk of the organism by eliminating one means of destroying it. In survival tests this organism may not show any advantage, but it must be considered at increased potential risk since it would be more difficult to remove. In contrast, the introduction of a gene for resistance to an antibiotic that is no longer used, because of natural resistance, would not change the relative risk to humans.

Assessment of Survival and Spread of the Extrachromosomal Elements

These studies should evaluate the potential for exchange of the designated cloned trait with other naturally occurring organisms sharing the environment [8,13,18,32,33]. If the cloning vehicle transfers to an endogenous

Table 3.5. The "Top Ten" Laboratory-Acquired Infections, 1930–1974

Infection	No. of Cases	No. of Deaths
Brucellosis	420	5
Q fever	280	1
Hepatitis	268	3
Typhoid fever	258	20
Tularaemia	225	2
Tuberculosis	194	4
Dermatomycosis	162	0
Venezuelan equine encephalitis	146	1
Psittacosis	116	10
Coccidioidomycosis	93	2
Total	2,168	48

From Collins [6], with permission.

Note: Not included are 113 cases of haemorrhagic fever contracted from wild rodents in one laboratory in Russia in 1962 [11a].

microorganism in that environment, it will have a greater survival advantage. This is particularly relevant in considering normal human skin and gut flora. Such studies should be done initially in vitro and then in animals or under environmental conditions as they pertain to the host organism. We and others have performed these kinds of experiments for transfer of genetic elements in sewage [13,26] and in the gut of man and animals [1–3,9, 11–17,19,20,22,29,30,35]. No colonization of mouse or human gut was found using a debilitated *E. coli* × 1776 or an *E. coli* K12 [14,15,17], *E. coli* K12 can survive for periods of days in the gut [1,19,30], and transfer of plasmids to endogenous hosts can occur [1,19,29]. Gut colonization was observed with wild type *E. coli*, where transfer of plasmid genes was readily demonstrated [12]. Decreasing microbial competition can improve transfer in vivo [3,11,17,20]. Transfer is greater in germ-free than in normal animals [11,15,17,19]. Antibiotic therapy, using a drug for which resistance is specified by the plasmid, gives advantage to the emergence of new transconjugants [3,19]. To avoid transfer, nontransferable, nonmobilizable genetic vehicles should be used. However, there may be future need for traits to be controllably exchanged within an environment. In this case, some knowledge of the spectrum of spread of a plasmid or transposon must be known. Differences in the extent of bacterial spread have led to the distinction between "permissive" and "nonpermissive" plasmids.

Table 3.6. Classification of Agents

Classification of bacterial agents

Class 1
All bacterial agents not included in higher classes according to "Basis for Agent Classifications"

Class 2
Actinobacillus — all species except *A. mallei*, which is in Class 3
Arizona hinshawii — all serotypes
Bacillus anthracis
Bordetella — all species
Borrelia recurrentis, B. Vincenti
Clostridium botulinum, Cl. chauvoei, Cl. haemolyticum, Cl. histolyticum, Cl. novyi, Cl. septicum, Cl. tetani
Corynebacterium diphtheriae, C. equi, C. haemolyticum, C. pseudotuberculosis, C. pyogenes, C. renale
Diplococcus (Streptococcus) pneumoniae
Erysipelothrix insidiosa
Escherichia coli — all enteropathogenic serotypes
Haemophilus ducreyi, H. influenzae
Herellea vaginicola
Klebsiella — all species and all serotypes
Leptospira interrogans — all serotypes
Listeria — all species
Mima polymorpha
Moraxella — all species
Mycobacteria — all species except those listed in Class 3
Mycoplasma — all species except *Mycoplasma mycoides* and *Mycoplasma agalactiae*, which are in Class 5
Neisseria gonorrhoeae, N. meningitidis
Pasteurella — all species except those listed in Class 3
Salmonella — all species and all serotypes
Shigella — all species and all serotypes
Sphaerophorus necrophorus
Staphylococcus aureus
Streptobacillus moniliformis
Streptococcus pyogenes
Treponema caratcum, T. pallidum, and *T. pertenue*
Vibrio fetus, V. comma, including biotype El Tor, and *V. parahemolyticus*

Class 3
Actinobacillus mallei
Bartonella — all species
Brucella — all species
Francisella tularensis
Mycobacterium avium, M. bovis, M. tuberculosis
Pasteurella multocida type B ("buffalo" and other foreign virulent strains)
Pseudomonas pseudomallei
Yersenia pestis

continued

Table 3.6. (Continued)

Classification of fungal agents

Class 1
All fungal agents not included in higher classes according to "Basis for Agent Classifications"

Class 2
Actinomycetes (including *Nocardia* species and *Actinomyces* species and *Arachnia propionica*)
Blastomyces dermatitidis
Cryptococcus neoformans
Paracoccidioides brasiliensis

Class 3
Coccidioides immitis
Histoplasma capsulatum
Histoplasma capsulatum var. *duboisii*

Classification of parasitic agents

Class 1
All parasitic agents not included in higher classes according to "Basis for Agent Classifications"

Class 2
Endamoeba histolytica
Leishmania sp.
Naegleria gruberi
Toxoplasma gondii
Toxocara canis
Trichinella spiralis
Trypanosoma cruzi

Class 3
Schistosoma mansoni

Classification of rickettsial and chlamydial agents

Class 1
includes all rickettsial and chlamydial agents not included in higher classes according to "Basis for Agent Classifications"

Class 2
Lymphogranuloma venereum agent

Class 3
Psittacosis Ornithosis Trachoma group of agents
Rickettsia — all species except *Vole rickettsia* when used for transmission or animal inoculation experiments

From the Department of Health, Education and Welfare [7].

Note: This classification does not include strictly animal pathogens.

A Public Health Service permit is required to import any agent or to transfer within the United States any agent imported under permit.

Table 3.7. Potential Secondary Effects of Introduced
Traits That Could Affect Human Health

Interference with body processes
  Metabolism
  Wound healing
  Host defenses
    immunologic
    cellular
    interference with phagocytosis
    increased survival against body defenses
  Growth and development (e.g., sexual)

Tropism for certain human tissues

Toxicity — skin; internal organs
  Accumulation of toxic by-products
  Release of known toxins

Create resistant or hard-to-treat infections

Diarrheal syndromes

Neurologic abnormalities — result of extracellular products

Cancer
  Production of growth factors
  Production of Missense RNAs

RISK ASSESSMENT STUDIES
USING DIFFERENT MILIEUS

This section considers the evaluation of human risk potentials under controllable laboratory conditions. It is assumed that the possibility for infection rests on evidence that the organism survives in the environment and has contact with man. (These latter issues are discussed in chapters 6 and 8.)

Growth Requirements of Microorganisms

Studies in vitro could define the substrate requirements as well as optima for temperature, pH, oxygen requirement, and so on, of the organism as an initial means of evaluating how like or unlike the engineered organism is to the original host organism from which it was derived. The findings would assess whether the inserted DNA has in any way changed the basic nutritional and atmospheric constraints of the organism. If the organism shows changes, such an alteration could potentially affect its ability to survive in different human tissues.

Survival in Human Products

Since infection by these organisms would necessitate surviving in body materials (e.g., blood, urine, feces, and saliva), it would be useful to know whether the organism could, in fact, survive in these milieus and, if so, for how long. These kinds of studies can be done under defined laboratory conditions. We have tested the survival of organisms in a 10% (W/V) solution of feces [14,15,17]. These studies were performed with unaltered as well as sterilized (autoclaved) fecal material. From these results, we determined that certain antimicrobial factors were inherent in fecal debris, and others were related to intestinal flora. We also learned that the sampling of one individual was not enough, and that studies of fecal specimens from 6 10 individuals were needed to provide a range of survival potentials.

Samples from more than one individual should be used in testing survival in blood, urine, and saliva because of differences in antibacterial activities, trace elements, and other factors that can affect survival and persistence. These studies will, in fact, help to identify endogenous features of body products that may prevent or permit survival. In these studies, the test organism should be evaluated in comparison with the unaltered original host.

Survival and Infection Potential in Animals

Most of the pathogenic studies of microorganisms have been done in animals, chiefly guinea pigs, mice, and some primates [6] (Table 3.8).

These studies have looked at the relative dose of an organism to cause infection (or death) in animals under different conditions and routes of entry. The results have then been translated into an infectious or lethal dose for man (Table 3.8).

It is most important to demonstrate that the organism under study has not changed its infectious dose. This can be confirmed by tests using the

Table 3.8. Microorganisms Required to Infect

Tuberculosis or BCG	10 guinea pig ID equals 1 ID[a] for man
Cholera	10^{11} vibrios for dog; 10^4 for man
Q fever	One organism for guinea pig or man
Scrub typhus	1 mouse ID equals 1 human ID
Tularaemia	10 organisms for mice, monkey, or man
Typhoid fever	10^{11} bacilli for chimpanzee; 10^8 or ^{9} for man

Adapted from Collins [6].

[a]ID = Infective Dose

unengineered control organism and the previous test animal. These kinds of studies, based on previously used animal models, permit comparative use of all previously obtained data such as infection rate and pathogenicity of the organism.

Risk Assessment in Humans

Experiments performed to assess risks in humans should focus on previous animal models. For direct tests in humans, the organisms could be tested for their ability to colonize the gut or skin, although such studies could be limited to those expected to have this potential. Our studies looking at the survival of bioengineered organisms in the gut of animals and man have shown that even naturally acquired *E. coli* had difficulty in colonizing the intestinal tract of man; and if they were debilitated, as in the case of *E. coli* K12, they were unable to colonize in the natural gut environment. However, these same organisms could colonize and persist in gut environments that were germ-free [17,21]. This finding highlighted and distinguished between those traits that were essential for growth of the organism and for intestinal colonization, and those traits that were needed to compete with other organisms or in environments altered by the growth of other organisms.

Other human studies could examine disease potential in nonhuman primates or human volunteers [4,5]. These are costly, could be hazardous, and probably are not necessary if prior studies are performed and organisms known to be nonpathogenic are used. Assessment in humans may only be needed if the organisms are shown to be altered vis à vis previous animal tests and/or able to persist in human products.

As an alternative to studies in man, there are certain in vitro tissue culture systems that might be applicable as a means of assessing human infection potential. Studies using tissue culture-grown human uroepithelial cells [27], human intestinal endothelial cells [34], human nasopharyngeal mucosa [31,36], fibrin-platelet matrices [28], human red cells [25], and other similar systems have demonstrated the ability of bacteria isolated from infections of these tissues to adhere to or interact with these cells when propagated in tissue culture. There appears to be a difference between naturally occurring pathogens and nonpathogens, based on the tissue culture results. These findings suggest assays in vitro for assessing the ability of engineered organisms to adhere to particular human tissues and to propagate — both necessary requirements for infection. Comparative studies using the engineered and nonengineered isogenic strains have potential importance in assessing pathogenicity. Additional studies of known pathogens and nonpathogens are needed, but these methodologies are in the process of evaluation and use and appear to provide a valuable alternative assay in vitro for assessing survival and pathogenicity in vivo. If reproducible values can be attained, direct studies in humans may not be needed.

Summary

By a combination of tests in vitro and in vivo in animals and humans, a thorough assessment of the organism for its survival and infection potential for man can be obtained. The potential risk to man resides firmly in the ability of these organisms to survive in the natural environment. In instances where one would want the organism to persist for hours or days, but not years, it is important to include characteristics that allow man to destroy the organism or that cause self-destruction. If an organism is to become fully established as a part of the ecosystem, it is important to see what happens to that ecosystem, in particular the other microorganisms sharing the environment, in reference to potential harm to humans. Most of these studies outlined can be done under laboratory conditions.

MONITORING OF HUMANS FOR EXPOSURE TO ORGANISMS RELEASED INTO THE ENVIRONMENT

It may be useful to survey the environment regularly for the appearance of the engineered organism, especially in regard to humans. Since the principal route of entry would be the skin, oropharynx, or gastrointestinal tract, assay systems for recovering the organism from these areas can be derived. For this purpose, a relatively unique biochemical or physical trait would be required in order to distinguish the engineered organism and its cloned gene from other natural organisms present. If there is concern about physiological changes secondary to release of products into the bloodstream, appropriate tests could be performed, including a search for antibodies to the organism or to its expressed product. These kinds of studies, however, appear difficult and cumbersome, and it is unclear whether they are even feasible or meaningful.

SUMMARY

The risk of exposure or harm of engineered organisms to humans should begin with an examination of the organism itself and its ability to survive in particular environments in which man directly interacts. This chapter has outlined a stepwise approach, which begins with the concept that the organism initially is developed in the laboratory from a naturally occurring organism. Knowing the original organism greatly aids in assessing its environmental niche and potential exposure to man. We can set up a series of probabilities for survival of the organism as it moves from ideal laboratory

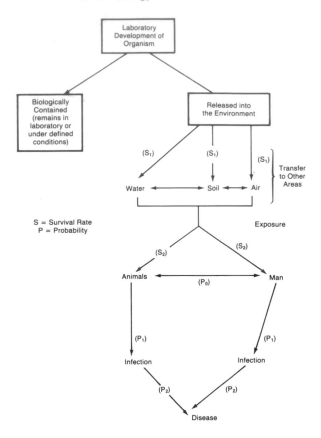

Figure 3.1. Risk evaluation approach.

conditions into different environmental areas (Fig. 3.1). If we know the survival potential in these areas, then we can begin to assess the relative exposure risks to humans. No exposure, of course, means no health risk. Based on the findings in the environment, we can move to studies of the organism's ability to survive in human body by-products and to colonize and cause infection in animals. Studies of the ability to propagate on human tissues in vitro may be a useful alternative to direct studies in man. The total evaluation should be based on the relative frequencies of each event tested in known, assessed models, using appropriate control organisms.

The kinds of experiments outlined here can feasibly be performed under experimentally controlled conditions. The data that arise should be statistically significant and useful in assessment, especially in view of all prior data available on the organism as an unengineered entity.

REFERENCES

1. Anderson, E. S. 1975. Viability of and transfer of a plasmid from *E. coli* K12 in the human intestine. *Nature* 255:502–504.
2. Anderson, J. D. 1975. Factors that may prevent transfer of antibiotic resistance between gram-negative bacteria in the gut. *J. Med. Microbiol.* 8:83–88.
3. Anderson, J. D., W. A. Gillespie, and M. H. Richmond. 1973. Chemotherapy and antibiotic resistance transfer between enterobacteria in the human gastrointestinal tract. *J. Med. Microbiol.* 6:461–473.
4. Beisel, W. R. 1983. Experimental respiratory tract infections in nonhuman primates. In G. Keusch and T. Wadstrom (Eds.), *Experimental Bacterial and Parasitic Infections*, pp. 241–245.
5. Beisel, W. R. and W. S. Stokes. 1983. Experimental infections in primates and human volunteers. In G. Keusch and T. Wadstrom (Eds.), *Experimental Bacterial and Parasitic Infections*, pp. 11–15.
6. Collins, C. H. 1983. *Laboratory-acquired infections.* Butterworths, London.
7. Department of Health, Education and Welfare. 1976. *Classification of Etiologic Agents on the Basis of Hazard.* Atlanta: Author.
8. Dougan, G., J. H. Crosa, and S. Falkow. 1978. Mobilization of the *Escherichia coli* plasmid ColE1 (colicin E1) and ColE1 vectors used in recombinant DNA experiments. *J. Inf. Diseases* 137:676–680.
9. Freter, R. 1978. Possible effects of foreign DNA on pathogenic potential and intestinal proliferation of *Escherichia coli. J. Inf. Diseases* 127:624–628.
10. Johanson, W. G., A. K. Pierce, and J. P. Sanford. 1969. Changing pharyngeal bacterial flora of hospitalized patients. *New Engl. J. Med.* 281:1137–1140.
11. Lafont, J. P., A. Bree, and M. Plat. 1984. Bacterial conjugation in the digestive tracts of gnotoxenic chickens. *Appl. Environ. Microbiol.* 47:639–642.
11a. Kulagin, S. M., W. I. Fedorova, and E. S. Ketiladze. 1962. Laboratory outbreak of hemorrhagic fever with renal syndrome. *Zhurnal Mikrobiologii Epidemiologii Immunologii* 33:121–126.
12. Levine, M. H., J. B. Kaper, H. Lockman, R. E. Black, M. L. Clements, and S. Falkow. 1983. Recombinant DNA risk assessment studies in humans: Efficacy of poorly mobilizable plasmids in biologic containment. *J. Inf. Diseases* 148:699–709.
13. Levy, S. B. 1984. Survival of plasmids in *Escherichia coli.* In W. Arber, K. Illmensee, W. J. Peacock, and P. Starlinger (Eds.), *Genetic Manipulation: Impact on Man and Society.* International Council of Scientific Union Press, Miami, Fl., pp. 19–28.
14. Levy, S. B. and B. Marshall. Survival of *E. coli* host-vector systems in the human intestinal tract. *Recombinant DNA Tech. Bull.* 2:77–80.
15. Levy, S. B. and B. Marshall. 1981. Risk assessment studies of *E. coli* host-vector systems. *Recombinant DNA Tech. Bull.* 4:91–98.
16. Levy, S. D., N. Sullivan and S. L. Gorbach. 1978. Pathogenicity of conventional and debilitated *E. coli* K-12. *Nature* 274:395–396.
17. Levy, S. B., B. Marshall, A. Onderdonk, and D. Rowse-Eagle. 1980. Survival of *E. coli* host-vector systems in the mammalian intestine. *Science* 209:391–394.
18. Marshall, B. and S. B. Levy. 1980. Prevalence of amber suppressor-containing coliforms in the natural environment. *Nature* 286:524–525.
19. Marshall, B., S. Schluederberg, C. Tachibana, and S. B. Levy. 1981. Survival

and transfer in the human gut of poorly mobilizable (pBR322) and of transferable plasmids from the same carrier *E. coli*. *Gene 14*:145–154.

20. Myhal, M. L., D. C. Laux, and P. A. Cohen. 1982. Relative colonizing activities of human fecal and K12 strains of *Escherichia coli* in the large intestines of streptomycin-treated mice. *Eur. J. Clin. Microbiol. 1*:186–192.

21. Onderdonk, A., B. Marshall, R. Cisneros, and S. B. Levy. 1981. Competition between congenic *Escherichia coli* K-12 strains *in vivo*. *Inf. Immun. 32*:74–79.

22. Petrocheilou, V., J. Grinsted, and M. H. Richmond. 1976. R plasmid transfer *in vivo* in the absence of antibiotic selection pressure. *Antimicrobiol. Agents Chem. 10*:753–761.

23. Pike, R. M. 1979. Laboratory-associated infections: Incidence, fatalities, causes and prevention. *Am. Rev. Microbiol. 33*:41–66.

24. Pike, R. M., S. E. Sulkin, and M. L. Schulze. 1965. Continuing importance of laboratory-acquired infections. *Am. J. Pub. Health 55*:190–199.

25. Ravdin, J. I. and R. L. Guerrant. 1981. Role of adherence in cytopathogenic mechanisms of *Entamoeba histolytica*. *J. Clin. Invest. 68*:1305–1313.

26. Sagik, B. P., C. A. Sorber, and B. E. Moore. 1981. The survival of EK1 and EK2 systems in sewage treatment plant models. In S. B. Levy, R. C. Clowes, and E. L. Koenig (Eds.), *Molecular Biology, Pathogenicity and Ecology of Bacterial Plasmids*. Plenum, New York, pp. 449–460.

27. Sandberg, T., K. Stenqvist, and C. Svanborg-Eden. 1979. Effects of subminimal inhibitory concentrations of ampicillin, chloramphenicol and nitrofurantoin on the attachment of *Escherichia coli* to human uroepithelial cells in vitro. *Rev. Inf. Diseases 1*:838–844.

28. Scheld, W. M., O. Zak, K. Vosbeck, and M. A. Sande. 1981. Bacterial adhesion in the pathogenesis of infective endocarditis. *J. Clin. Invest. 68*:1381–1384.

29. Smith, H. W. 1969. Transfer of antibiotic resistance from animal and human strains of *Escherichia coli* to resident *E. coli* in the alimentary tract of man. *Lancet 1*:1174–1176.

30. Smith, H. W. 1975. Survival of orally administered *E. coli* K12 in the alimentary tract of man. *Nature 255*:500–502.

31. Stephens, D. S., L. H. Hoffman, and Z. A. McGee. 1983. Interaction of *Neisseria meningitidis* with human nasopharyngeal mucosa: Attachment and entry into columnar epithelial cells. *J. Inf. Diseases 148*:369–376.

32. Stotzky, G. and H. Babich. 1984. Fate of genetically engineered microbes in natural environments. *Recombinant DNA Tech. Bull. 7*:163–188.

33. Stotzky, G. and V. N. Krasowsky. 1981. Ecological factors that affect the survival, establishment, growth and genetic recombination of microbes in natural habitats. In S. B. Levy, R. C. Clowes, and E. L. Koenig (Eds.), *Molecular Biology, Pathogenicity and Ecology of Bacterial Plasmids*. Plenum, New York, pp. 31–42.

34. Vosbeck, K. and U. Huber. 1982. An assay for measuring specific adhesion of an *Escherichia coli* strain to tissue culture cells. *Eur. J. Clin. Microbiol. 1*:22–28.

35. Williams, P. H. 1977. Plasmid transfer in the human alimentary tract. *FEMS Microbial. Lett. 2*:91–95.

36. Woods, D. E., D. C. Straus, W. G. Johanson, and J. R. Bass. 1981. Role of salivary protease activity in adherence of gram-negative bacilli to mammalian buccal epithelial cells in vivo. *J. Clin. Invest. 68*:1435–1440.

4

Human Exposure to Viruses and Effects Assessment

Alfred Hellman

The fundamental properties of animal viruses play a significant role in the determination of their potential risk with respect to environmental applications of biotechnology. Viruses multiply only within fully functional cells and are very fastidious in terms of the cells that they will infect. A very limited number of biochemical functions are under their control, and viruses are virtually totally dependent on the cell's synthesizing capabilities for multiplication.

Many viral diseases have had a major impact on man. Over the past 30 years, viruses have served as models by which many basic biological problems have been resolved. Resolution of these problems has led to fundamental understanding and considerable progress in the detection of viruses and their components once they have infected living cells.

The currently envisioned applications of viruses in biotechnology, that is, as vectors for repair genes, as subviral vaccines, and in agriculture, suggest that they will not be a major risk factor. Risk assessment methodologies can be evaluated by discussing the properties of human viruses and their potential once they enter a viable cell. It will become clear that there are numerous ways of determining whether viral infection has occurred, and that viruses can be engineered to "self-destruct."

Though in nature viruses undergo a high degree of mutability, established and developing technologies increasingly permit their detection in a variety of environments. The technology that permits the transfer of genetic information among species should effectively allow for the rapid and specific detection of such transposition. This is the case, since we know what genetic information and immunological responses to look for.

In the absence of man-made limitations on viral mutation and spread, natural viral mutations have been observed over the centuries. Even so, nature has limited the establishment of significant deleterious genetic information in the species. Through the tools of modern biotechnology, we can design the introduction of genetic information in ways that will assure the safety of the viral application.

BACKGROUND

Animal Viruses as Entities

Structure and Chemical Composition. In rather fundamental terms, a virus is a piece of nucleic acid, either ribonucleic acid (RNA) or deoxyribonucleic acid (DNA), enclosed in a protein coat (nonenveloped viruses) or a protein coat and a lipid envelope. All known single- and multi-cell species, including man, carry viruses. Virus particles that have been isolated from their intracellular incubator can be regarded as inert biochemicals that have no independent replicative functions, unless they are reincorporated into a cell that has the capacity to provide those metabolic processes that permit the particle to reproduce itself.

The protein of the virus has several functions. It protects the nucleic acid of the virus so that the latter can faithfully act as a template for viral progeny. It protects the virus against detrimental environmental factors and serves as a protective shell that prevents nucleases (enzymes that break down nucleic acids) from destroying the virus during its course through the body prior to reaching appropriate cells in which the virus can replicate.

A second and highly significant function of the protein coat of nonenveloped viruses, relevant to risk, is that it controls the host range of the virus. In other words, the protein limits the entrance of nucleic acid to only those cells to which the protein can adsorb by specific virus-cell receptor sites. In the absence of such a site, which may be visualized as a lock and key, it has been demonstrated that virus attachment is prevented. In addition, the protein of the virus in most instances elicits one or several specific immunological responses that are protective for the host and serve as a means for detecting the presence of viral infection [1].

The quantity of nucleic acid that a specific virus such as poliovirus, poxvirus, or influenza virus contains determines the amount of genetic information that the virus can transmit. It also determines how much metabolic help the virus requires from its host (i.e., the cell in which it replicates). For example, poliovirus can code for no more than approximately 4 to 8 average-size proteins [2]. Herpes virus, which is approximately 100 times larger than poliovirus, codes for many more viral-directed proteins. Such proteins serve as the structural elements of the virus, and some have very specialized functions [3]. For example, certain proteins called enzymes provide advantages for the survivability of the virus as well as for reducing the requirements for specific host metabolic processes. Knowledge of viral genomic composition can be utilized effectively to construct viruses, by genetic engineering, that are even more limited in their host range. In cases where viruses are well characterized, there is the potential for introduction of self-destructive mechanisms at the enzyme level. For example, the presence of RNA-dependent DNA polymerase enzyme (reverse transcriptase) in animal RNA tumor viruses is being explored as a vehicle for the integration of beneficial genetic information into animals and humans.

In addition to significant diversity in the amount of nucleic acid that a particular type of virus contains, the nucleic acid can be either single- or double-stranded RNA or DNA. The single-stranded RNA viruses, such as poliovirus, RNA tumor virus, and others, serve as direct templates in the host for translation into progeny virus and are called positive-stranded viruses [4,5]. Viral RNAs that need to be transcribed into positive strands, as is the case with many of the viruses that cause encephalitis, are negative-stranded viruses. The requirement for transcribing negative strands into positive strands may be used in the construction of viral properties that limit the virus's ability to replicate in the absence of a polymerase enzyme.

Although most viral RNA consists of unbroken strands of nucleic acid, some viral genomes, such as the influenza, lassa, and arboviruses, consist of segmented RNA molecules. A consequence of such segmentation is that highly efficient genetic recombination can occur by random reassortment. Influenza viruses use this property very effectively in their continued genetic variation. Minor influenza variations bring about epidemics every 1 or 2 years, while major antigenic variations cause pandemics every 10 to 15 years.

Mechanism of Infection. It has been well established that risk of viral infection is based on some or all of the following factors [9]:

1. The number and severity of infections that occur in the population.
2. The physiological factors that modify infection.
3. Dose of virus required to cause an infection.
4. Degree of horizontal transmission of the agent.
5. Secretion of the agent in feces, urine, and saliva.
6. Degree of viremia (i.e., dissemination of viruses by the blood).
7. Propensity of the virus to remain in the population in a subclinical form.
8. Mutability of the virus in nature.
9. Specific requirements of the virus for host factors that permit infection to occur.
10. Host range.

Even though these factors are recognized as influencing risk, many are not well understood.

Viruses survive by the fact that they interact with cells in which they can replicate or integrate, that is, become a component of the cell's genome. Since viruses only represent a hazard in those situations in which they find a suitable living cell system in which they can integrate and/or replicate, it is important to gain a fundamental understanding of this process. Intervention in this process by a variety of natural and man-made methods can either enhance or prevent such infections from occurring.

Once virus receptor and cell receptor find complementation, adsorption of virus to the cell surface can occur. The second step of this process, specific receptor molecular interaction, is highly animal-, organ-, and cell-specific. For example, mouse tumor viruses only infect mice of specific genetic composition and only cells of certain mouse organs, such as the thymus, spleen, or lymph nodes. In man, poliovirus only adsorbs to cell receptors in the central nervous system and the intestinal tract that are specifically coded for by genetic information contained in chromosome 19. Cells that have such receptor sites frequently have as many as 100,000 sites per cell for a particular virus type. This obviously provides the potential for genetic recombination to occur between similar viruses entering one cell.

In vitro, these early stages of virus infection are highly inefficient, since adsorption may occur at cell receptor sites at which penetration cannot occur. In addition, the viral genome may be damaged by cell membrane nucleases, or the penetrating virus may not be released from the phagocytic vacuole. This suggests that significant numbers of virus are necessary to produce infection in vivo, pointing toward a reduced risk potential.

The virus protein plays a major role in the ability of the virus to traverse and survive the external environment and to locate proper cell attachment sites. The protein protects the virus and limits the number of animals, including man, that it can infect (host range). For some viruses, the host range can be broadened significantly by removal of the viral protein. By a process called transfection, performed under stringent laboratory conditions, either viral or cellular naked nucleic acids can be transmitted into cells [7].

Though transfection demonstrates the existence of a potential hazard, it also suggests a rather minimal likelihood for such an event to occur. Naked nucleic acids of such viruses as herpes, arbo, polio, and certain upper respiratory viruses are infectious if they can gain entrance to cells. Therefore, viruses with RNA that can act directly as messenger RNA without being transcribed from negative to positive strands have an advantage in this process.

In all cases, naked nucleic acids, although having increased host range, are significantly less infectious, by a factor of one thousand to one million, than the whole virus particles from which they are extracted. Two important reasons for this reduced infectivity are that the nucleic acid is (1) very inefficiently adsorbed onto the cell, and (2) readily degraded by enzymes within the cell. Interestingly, naked nucleic acid does have a much greater degree of stability in ambient environments. Nucleic acid, although highly susceptible to nucleases, has been shown to remain infectious for many days under such adverse conditions as high temperature and low humidity, and in the presence of neutralizing antibody. Thus, viral protein represents the most labile component of the virus.

Viral Integration or Replication. The most frequently observed virus–cell interactions are either lytic infections of the cell, where the virus replicates in the cell and produces cell disruption, or a transformational interaction. In transformation the viral genome is integrated into the host genome and produces a permanent alteration in the cells. Integration may lead to either cell transformation, which results in changes in cell morphology or growth, or a latent state. All transformation is seen with tumor virus, where either leukemias, lymphomas, or sarcomas eventually become evident, whereas latent state is seen in herpes virus infection, where pathology frequently is expressed only when the host is stressed. Other viruses, the so-called slow viruses, may infect an individual and not manifest pathology for as long as 20 to 40 years [6].

Viral Transmission

Survival in the Environment. Whole viruses within cells or surrounded by other natural materials may retain infectivity for up to 24 hours or longer. Exceptions exist, such as baculoviruses, which survive considerably longer and are considered to be environmentally stable when within an occlusion body. It is normal for viruses to be transmitted within protective protein-aceous substances such as cells, saliva, urine, feces, and blood serum. Survivability is influenced by such factors as UV rays from sunlight, pH, temperature, humidity, and other environmental stresses that act on the protein of the virus, thereby preventing it from participating in the process of infection.

Routes of Infection. Numerous routes of viral infection have been recognized. Frequently the most efficient route of infection is via the mucous membranes of the respiratory tract. However, recent studies have suggested that even respiratory viruses may more effectively cause upper respiratory disease by transmission via direct contact rather than inhalation [8]. A virus may also gain entrance by ingestion and subsequent adsorption via mucous membranes of the gastrointestinal and genitourinary tracts. Direct inoculation of the virus may occur by sexual transmission and fecal-oral dissemination. The most direct and efficient route in terms of number of infectious virus particles required for infection is inoculation into the skin or bloodstream. However, this does not occur frequently except where specific insects act as reservoirs and vectors for the virus (i.e., arboviruses).

Because it is composed of several keratinized, nonviable cell layers, intact skin is a formidable protective layer for the body. The mucous membranes are also protective, since they are continually in contact with many fluids that contain both specific and nonspecific antiviral factors. There is no indication that a viral disease manifests itself in different pathologies when introduced by abnormal routes into the body. However, if a particular virus, such as one that ultimately infects the central nervous system, gains access to cells of that system without traversing through other parts of the body, there is less opportunity for the host to mount a defense and therefore decreased opportunity for early detection to occur.

Host Range. It is critically important to recognize that, in general, viruses have a limited range of animals that they will infect. This host range restriction is highly significant when considering the potential risk of a viral agent to humans. This phenomenon also permits a means of assessing human exposure.

Viral Mutation and Recombination. Spontaneous mutations occur continually in the course of viral multiplication. Some of these mutations may be lethal to the virus while others permit the virus to adapt to conditions under which they replicate. Frequently, science has taken advantage of mutations to develop attenuated viruses that have and still are being used as live vaccines.

In nature, viruses should be regarded as a genetically heterogeneous population. They may contain mutants produced at an average rate of one per million organisms. This should be taken into consideration for risk evaluation since the very modifications that now can be performed in the laboratory may have been occurring for millions of years without apparent long-term, harmful effects to plants, animals, or humans.

The knowledge gained from natural mutation and the culturing of such viruses has provided an approach for introducing self-destructive characteristics into the virus. For example, it is possible to select or engineer a virus that will not replicate at the normal body temperature of 36–37 degrees C, but will grow at lower temperatures. Other viral mutations that have been used to advantage are drug resistance, host range, enzyme deficiencies, and so-called hot mutants. Another type of virus that has been frequently encountered in most families of viruses is a defective virus. These viruses cannot grow by themselves but need a helper virus to replicate. Defective viruses can readily be used as antigens without significant hazard that they will infect and replicate in the host. This is an example of yet another natural phenomenon that can be exploited in the use of viruses for beneficial functions.

Viruses as Genetic Vectors. The advent of recombinant DNA technology has raised the hope that it can be applied to correct human genetic deficiency diseases. This possibility has led to a search for vehicles that can introduce such genetic information into the patient. One such technique currently under active investigation is the use of the RNA tumor virus. The thought is that the transforming genome of the virus could be deleted, permitting the genetic information for correcting the genetic deficiency to be introduced into the virus. Since such viruses have an RNA dependent DNA polymerase, they could infect appropriate patient cells and integrate the medical gene into the patient genome. Future therapeutic applications in individuals who have genetic deficiencies, such as the capacity to produce insulin and growth hormones, as well as immunological deficiencies may become feasible. Similarly, by using a vaccine strain of vaccinia virus engineered to carry genetic information for stimulating antibodies to any number of human viral diseases, a single inoculation could serve multiple purposes, without the risk of introducing competent viruses that might back-mutate to a virulent form [10].

VIRUSES AS POTENTIAL PESTICIDES

Certain insect viruses (baculoviruses) are registered by the Environmental Protection Agency as effective biological pesticides. The release of such biological agents into the environment raises some safety questions. Unfortunately we have only a limited body of knowledge about the molecular, cellular, and antigenic properties and host range of these large DNA viruses.

The control of cotton bollworm and tobacco budworm by baculovirus has permitted epidemiological evaluations to be performed on individuals who manufacture and handle these agents, as well as on persons who apply them agriculturally. To this date no recognized pathological or serological conversion has been observed. Additionally in vivo pathogenicity tests have been performed on mammals, avians, and amphibians [11].

It should, however, be recognized that our meager understanding of these complex viruses diminishes the utility of these observations. Baculoviruses have a uniquely environmentally stable form — the occlusion body. The virus is occluded within a phosphoprotein crystal matrix that is responsible for horizontal transmission and not found in vertebrates. In this form, baculoviruses can be transmitted over great distances and can persist for extended time periods. Though baculoviruses are not known to be human pathogens, cell culture studies indicate that they are quite capable of entering vertebrate cells, uncoating, and perhaps undergoing some limited replication. Penetration appears to be temperature-independent, occurring in the cold. There are also recent data that associate a certain neurological disease with scientists who work with viruses of fruit trees.

Not only baculoviruses but also bacteriophages are being considered for control of plant pathogens. Many of the agents used as microbial pesticides are extremely poorly characterized, and their taxonomy is poorly elucidated. Because many of these viruses have no appropriate in vitro cultivation system, analyses by restriction enzymes are difficult to do. There is, however, available evidence of DNA homology (over 30%) between poliovirus and cowpea mosaic virus, a divided-genome single-stranded RNA virus that uses a replication scheme very similar to poliovirus [16]. An in-depth understanding of these agents will provide more assurance to proceed in their application (potentially as modified by genetic engineering) for agricultural purposes. High priority should be given to studies of the basic virology, genetics, and molecular biology of these agents as well as any others contemplated as biological pesticides.

HOST RESPONSE, RISK, AND DETECTION METHODOLOGY

When viral infection occurs, the host responds at a number of levels. A brief discussion of these responses will provide a clearer understanding of how they may be utilized to detect infection.

Histological and Pathological Responses. The most readily observed effects of a lytic viral infection are the cytopathic effects. Frequently, the nucleus becomes pyknotic, and cells in culture detach from their adhering surfaces and round up. These degenerative changes are brought about by a series of events. In some viral infections, they are due to proteins that are synthesized by the cell soon after viral infection and are under viral control. In other instances, these responses may be due to components of the infecting virus. Inhibition of host-directed cellular synthesis, which occurs in poliovirus and vaccinia virus infection, may account for the histological changes. Certain genetic expressions regulated by the host also frequently are altered and new functions are initiated, such as the synthesis of interferon. It also has been suggested that many cellular DNA functions, which are normally not expressed, may be initiated after viral infection. These all permit a means of diagnosis of viral infection.

Immunological and Cellular Modification. Certain antigenic changes can occur at the surface of infected cells. The presence of these altered surface antigens frequently triggers the host to initiate a defensive immune response targeted at eliminating the infected cells.

At times, certain viruses will alter the host range characteristics of the cell. This helper effect, imparted by the first virus, most likely occurs because the first virus induces certain functions in the cell that permit the second virus to enter and replicate. This phenomenon has been demonstrated primarily in animal systems and in tissue culture, but should still be considered in the overall context of risk assessment and detection of viral infection.

Host Physiology. To some extent, the severity of a viral infection is dependent on the physiological status of the host. Such factors as age, sex, hormonal balance, nutrition, secondary infection, and race, among others, influence whether the individual will be infected, and the severity of infection. Consequently, in assessing risk, the question of the groups at risk or sensitive subpopulations must be considered and taken advantage of as a means of detection.

Epidemiology. Our understanding of the epidemiology of human viral infection has been well documented over the past 40 to 50 years. Dissemination, severity, and incidence are unquestionably dependent on the factors discussed thus far, namely:

1. Continued presence in the population, primarily in subclinical form.
2. Virulence of the microorganism.
3. Route of infection.
4. Mutability of the virus.
5. Host range of the virus.
6. Host response by immunological and other host defenses.
7. Accessibility of an antibody to the infectious agent.

A brief epidemiological example of a few of these agents can be instructive.

Influenza infections of humans, particularly of the pandemic and epidemic type, have been documented over the past 95 years. Epidemics of this disease can occur at any time in the tropics, with epidemics recorded in the United States every month of the year. A significant reason for this occurrence is the fact that the virus has reservoirs in a variety of animal species and undergoes minor and major mutations continually. It is transmitted readily through the respiratory route by droplets containing high-titered virus, and thus gains access to susceptible cells. Frequently, 90% of an exposed population will experience clinical symptoms as a result of limited exposure to the virus. The lack of specific neutralizing antibodies permits the disease to manifest itself, and the development of antibodies permits detection of the virus and limits its spread.

Approximately 25% to 60% of those exposed become infected when a new strain of virus appears in the population. Secondary antigenic drifts usually occur in a specific strain, which cause a majority of antibody-negative individuals to develop clinical signs over the next 1 to 5 years. Additionally, some of the previously infected individuals can be reinfected due to their poor initial immune response or waning primary response. Once the majority of a population has been exposed and has developed immunity, new viral strains begin to emerge, and the cycle repeats itself [12].

The poxviruses, of which smallpox is the primary human disease, constitute another epidemiological example, but with an entirely different sequel. Man is the natural host, and transmission occurs primarily by person-to-person contact via the respiratory tract. The virus has remained quite stable over the years. Even though its presence as a major health problem has been documented, with epidemics occurring over the past 3,000 years, vaccination basically has eradicated the disease worldwide. An example of the severity of this type of disease in a virgin population was documented in 1721, when almost 50% of the Boston population became infected.

A brief discussion of the RNA tumor viruses is warranted, primarily because of their integration within the cell rather than any significant number of human malignancies attributable to this class of viruses. They are highly species-specific and are primarily transmitted via the animal genome, from mother to offspring (vertical).

In most instances they do not cause documented tumors in nature, except for cats, some mice, and some cattle. By very sensitive immunological and biochemical means, however, genomic components or whole viruses are found in all mammals, reptiles, and amphibians [13]. Since these viruses are transmitted vertically, they are not recognized as foreign antigens by the host, and antibodies are normally difficult to detect by immunological means. Recently, human T-cell lymphoma, a rare form of human malignancy, has been thought to be etiologically caused by an RNA tumor virus. It also has been suggested that a similar virus may be etiologically associated with Acquired Immune Deficiency Syndrome (AIDS).

EVALUATION OF DIAGNOSTIC METHODOLOGY

By virtue of the nature of viruses and the types of host responses that have been described, numerous methods for the diagnosis of viral presence, exposure, and disease are available. These tools include the microscopic observation of cytological changes brought about by certain viruses and immunological responses to infection.

Traditional methods for ascertaining the presence of viral information depend primarily on the host's immunological response. The commonly accepted serological techniques, such as complement fixation (CF), hemagglutination inhibition (HI), and viral neutralization (N), are still of significant diagnostic value today. However, these methodologies require that the virus replicate in the host and that the host in turn mount an immunological response. The CF test is particularly rapid and allows one to determine if a particular viral infection occurred recently. CF antibodies, however, decline more rapidly than specific neutralizing antibodies. Hemagglutination antibodies are quite specific and correlate well with neutralizing antibodies, but not all viruses elicit HI antibodies. On the other hand, N antibodies are quite specific, last a long time, and normally confer immunity to the host, although a conventional test for N antibody presence requires that the virus be grown in cell culture.

Newer immunological assays have evolved over the past several years. They include the enzyme-linked immunosorbent assay (ELISA) and the radioimmunoassay (RIA). These tests are dependent on colorimetric or isotopic detection and are much more sensitive. They are rapidly replacing the more traditional immunological means. In general, they do not require that the virus be isolated prior to confirming its presence in the host. However, a detailed antigenic understanding of the virus is required.

Other sensitive immunological techniques utilize immunofluorescence, which detects the presence of small numbers of viruses in cells. This is a highly specific and sensitive test for certain viruses that can provide reliable data in less than one day. However, this method of diagnosis still requires meticulous preparation of reagents to achieve the sensitivity and specificity that the technology is capable of delivering.

Recently developed monoclonal antibodies make diagnosis by immunological means highly specific and quite sensitive [14]. This technology has led to an avalanche of diagnostic kits, and it permits the detection of viruses and small components of viruses to an extreme degree of specificity. Monoclonal antibodies represent a major breakthrough in the diagnosis of very early events in viral infection.

The ability to dissect the virus nucleic acid by enzymes, as used in genetic engineering, has led to the evolution of a diagnostic tool, the DNA probe [15], to detect the presence of a small portion of one viral nucleic acid in one cell. As this technology develops, it should be feasible to determine the presence of even a small fragment of a virus, at times during the viral infectious cycle prior to replication. One should also be able to detect the presence of viral nucleic acid in air samples. As isotopic labeling techniques become more sensitive, DNA and RNA hybridization probes could be powerful tools for routine detection of nucleic acid sequences introduced into human and animal DNA. It must be emphasized, however, that this technology is still evolving and at this time does not have the discriminatory capabilities to identify small quantities of foreign nucleic acid in the presence of large amounts of native DNA. As in most immunological diagnostic tests for which the antigenicity of the virus needs to be known, the molecular biology of the virus in question must be well understood in order to effectively apply nucleic acid hybridization probe technology.

NEEDED RESEARCH

The following areas merit attention in future research:

- Currently available DNA and RNA hybridization probe technology could be improved. In particular, enhancing its capacity to discriminate between natural and exogenous nucleic acids would be useful.
- Sensitive nonradioactive labeling technology needs to be developed for routine use as a diagnostic tool in nucleic acid probe analysis.
- An in-depth understanding of biology, virology, genetics, and molecular biology must be gained for those viruses, such as baculovirus and certain phages, being considered for use as pesticides in the environment.
- An understanding of the antigenic components of biological pesticides needs to be obtained, particularly those that may elicit specific immunological responses in mammals. Once identified and isolated, such antigens can be used in the development of specific diagnostic reagents for retrospective epidemiology and environmental monitoring.

REFERENCES

1. Dimmock, N. J. 1982. Initial stages in infection with animal viruses. *J. Gen. Virol. 59*:1.
2. Adler, C. J., M. Elzinga, and E. Wimmer. 1983. The genome-linked protein of picornaviruses. VIII. Complete amino acid sequence of poliovirus VPg and carboxyterminal analysis of its precursor, P3-9. *J. Gen. Virol. 64*:349.
3. Lee, G. T., M. F. Y. Para, and P. G. Spear. 1982. Location of the structural genes for glycoprotein gD and gE and for other polypeptides in the S component of herpes simplex virus type 1 DNA. *J. Gen. Virol. 43*:41.
4. Weiss, R., N. Teich, and H. Varmus, Eds. 1982. *Tumor Viruses.* Cold Spring Harbor Lab, Cold Spring Harbor, N.Y.
5. Putnak, J. R. and B. A. Phillips. 1981. Picornaviral structure and assembly. *Microbiol. Rev. 45*:287.
6. Simons, K., H. Garoff, and A. Helenius. 1982. How an animal virus gets into and out of its host cell. *Sci. Am. 246*:58.
7. Colburn, H. H., C. B. Talmadge, and T. D. Gindhart. 1983. Transfer of sensitivity to tumor promoters by transfection of DNA from sensitive to insensitive mouse JB6 epidermal cells. *Mol. & Cell. Biol. 3*:1182.

8. Beisel, W. 1985. Personal communication. Johns Hopkins University, Baltimore, Md.
9. West, D. L., D. R. Twardzik, R. W. McKinney, W. E. Barkley, and A. Hellman. 1980. *Identification, Analysis and Control of Biohazards in Viral Cancer Research Laboratory Safety.* Academic Press, New York.
10. *Genetic Engineering News, 1985*, 5(3):17.
11. Valli, V. E., J. C. Cunningham, and B. M. Arif. 1976. Tests demonstrating the safety of baculovirus of spruce budworm to mammals and birds. In *Proceedings of the First International Colloquium on Invertebrate Pathology.* Queen's University, Kingston, Ontario, Canada, pp. 445-446.
12. Dowdle, N. R., M. T. Coleman, and M. B. Gregg. 1974. Natural history of influenza type A in the U.S. 1957-1972. *Prog. Med. Virol. 17:91.*
13. Bishop, J. M. Cellular oncogenes and retroviruses. 1983. *Ann. Rev. Biochem.* 52:301.
14. Fazekes de St., S. Groth, and D. Scheidegger. 1980. Production of monoclonal antibodies: Strategy and tactics. *J. Immunol. Meth. 35:1.*
15. Alwine, J. J., D. J. Kemp, and G. R. Stark. 1977. Method for detection of specific RNA's in agarose gels by transfer to diazobenzyloxymethyl paper and hybridization with DNA probes. *Proc. Natl. Acad. Sci. U.S.A.* 74:5350.
16. Franssen, H., J. Leumissen, R. Goldbach, G. Lomonossoff, and D. Zimmerman. 1984. Homology sequences in cowpea mosaic virus and poliovirus. *EMBO* 3(4):855-861.

5

Ecological Consequence Assessment: Effects of Bioengineered Organisms

John Cairns, Jr. and James R. Pratt

This chapter critically reviews methods for ecological assessment and evaluates these methods as tools for monitoring effects of genetically altered microorganisms on ecological processes and structures. Ecosystems have two fundamental properties: they are comprised of structures, and these structures perform particular functions. The relationship between structure and function is not clear and has led to arguments concerning structural relationships between species diversity and community stability [23]. Rather than studying the bewildering array of species that literally number in the millions, many ecologists direct their attention toward summarizing important biochemical transformations. This approach, known as systems ecology, reduces the complexity of ecosystems to a few compartments where energy and nutrients may flow [22]. A simple compartment model for the flow of energy in an ecosystem is shown in Figure 5.1. Depending on how carefully one dissects the system of interest, however, the compartment model may become quite complex.

Three possible relationships exist between structure and function, and there is no general agreement as to the validity of each relationship.

1. Structure and function are intimately related; a change in one causes a concomitant change in the other.
2. System function is generally maintained over a wide range of conditions, and a great deal of functional redundancy occurs in the component biota. The structure of the system may change radically from day to day or from season to season, but the overall functioning of the system

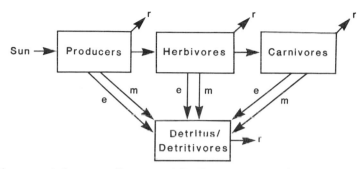

Key: r = respiration; e = egestion; m = mortality. The unlabeled arrows represent ingestion.

Figure 5.1. Simple compartment model of energy and carbon flow in a generalized ecosystem.

remains essentially constant. In this case, a change in structure that might be caused by an environmental disturbance might be confused with a normal internal cycle of component populations.

3. Broad physiological ranges of most organisms allow them to survive even though overall system function may be severely impaired. That is, the mere presence of particular organisms in an ecosystem may be a poor reflection of the functional state or potential of the system.

In case 1, the intimate relationship between system structure and function means that parameters reflective of each may be measured as an index of system health. In case 2, the ability of the system to maintain function in the face of changing structure may be considered evidence of the conservative nature of functional measurements, that is, system function may be maintained despite wholesale changes in the biotic structure. In this case, structural changes might be considered early warning signals of eventual system collapse. In case 3, the ability of organisms to maintain their biological integrity during disturbances can be interpreted as evidence of the conservative nature of structural measurements. That is, community or ecosystem structure may be maintained as an artifact of the physiological range of the component populations, though overall system functioning is severely impaired. Here structure is the more conservative variable, and it would be argued that measuring functional responses or attributes would provide greater early warning of adverse effects.

At the present time, regulatory agencies generally have taken an approach that protects system structure, usually by basing standards on the behavior of laboratory-tolerant species toward anthropogenic insults. In most ecosystems the types of organisms usually used for testing perform trivial functions. In aquatic ecosystems, the mass of carbon found in living tissue at any given time is generally less than 1% of the available carbon in the system [10]. Most of the remainder of this carbon, like carbon in many other ecosystems, is in the form of dead organic matter or detritus. Recycling of this dead organic material, chiefly by microbial species, provides a food source for a large number of species in the detritus food chain [21,31] and mineralizes and makes available inorganic materials (nitrogen, phosphorus, sulfur, and trace elements) previously bound in biomass and necessary for continued system function. Many ecologists believe that the maintenance of energy, carbon, and nutrient cycling processes is the fundamental characteristic of ecosystems. Others believe that the size, rate of growth, and diversity of natural populations are reflective of environmental conditions. In terms of maintenance of system function, the loss or gain of one or a few species is trivial as long as system function is maintained. Alternatively, many ecologists see the loss of a particular species as a loss of residual genetic diversity and, consequently, of evolutionary potential.

While it may be argued that changes in the composition of species at particular trophic levels (herbivores, carnivores) reflect changes in the system at lower levels, there is no doubt that the greatest amount of biomass and residual carbon is in the detrital compartment, at least in aquatic ecosystems [31]. The truly critical processes in most ecosystems occur in this compartment and result in the liberation of nutrients and the processing of dead material. In addition, bacterial decomposers are the mainstay of these processes and may be considered the most likely targets for adverse effects from genetically altered microorganisms [8]. A large number of other species have evolved to make use of the nutrients and materials in the detrital pool; for example, several tens of thousands of species of microorganisms either prey directly on bacteria in the sediments or use bacteria and the associated detritus as food sources. Photosynthetic microbial species, such as diatoms and other algae, also grow on surfaces and sediments and make direct use of the nutrient materials released during decomposition. Other more highly evolved species prey on the algae or bacterial grazers, and many juvenile insects feed directly on detritus and its associated microflora of bacteria. As one moves up the food chain, predators become less diverse but larger in size.

A number of methods are used to assess the structure and function of ecosystems. Approaches to assessing functional attributes rely on the measurement of rates of conversion of materials and the development of input–output models. Approaches to measuring system structure generally involve stratifying the component biota into categories based either on taxonomic relationships or location within the system. For example, a survey of an aquatic ecosystem might include specialists for sampling fish, microinvertebrates (insects, snails, worms), algae, and protozoa. For most structural surveys, "critter counting" is a must, as is taxonomic precision. In general, the smaller an organism, the less likely it is to be studied.

Evaluating the potential effects of biotechnology products is fundamentally different from evaluation of chemical effects. Because organisms are being introduced into the environment, it is necessary to understand their biology (especially their autoecology) in developing tests for potential effects. Introduced organisms, even those heavily modified, have the potential to survive and reproduce. Additionally, these organisms may be transported to other ecosystems either passively, by physical factors such as water and air movement, or by animal or human dispersal agents. One or a few founding individuals might then multiply and express some trait deleterious to the structure or function of the system. To a large extent, the probability of establishment of introduced, genetically altered species is related to the characteristics of the source species [18].

To utilize ecosystem assessments fully in examining the potential effects of genetically altered species, it is necessary to relate any phenomenon studied to the probable dose of foreign material. Estimates of this dose require knowledge of fate and transport effects and will assume that a suitable means is available for accurate detection of the transport rate in the area over which the material has spread. Ecological assessments of system structure and function probably will be used at two major points in the development and use of biotechnology products: during field trials, and for post hoc assessments of purported damage, as is now employed for pollution effects studies. In the latter case, it might be expected that ecological assessments would be used as environmental surveillance tools [15] to verify that no adverse effects had occurred. As with most scientific research, verification of a negative is very difficult. If testing procedures used for estimating the environmental effects of genetically altered species are sufficiently sophisticated, it should be possible to make comparable measurements in the field to verify whether novel organisms have, in fact, invaded an area and to measure the effects of this invasion on the resident biota.

AVAILABLE METHODS
IN ECOLOGICAL ASSESSMENT

Ecological assessment has at least two purposes in the regulation of biotechnology products (Fig. 5.2). In the first place, approximate model ecosystems (microcosms, mesocosms) should be designed for adequately evaluating potential adverse impacts before any such products are released into the environment. The form of these model ecosystems depends on the probable sites of impact and on the questions asked in the research program. For example, if the release site is in an effluent to an aquatic eco-

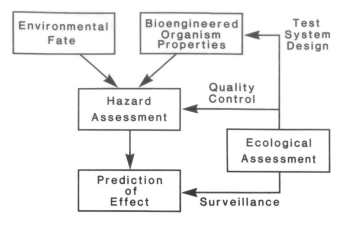

Figure 5.2. Place of ecological assessment in the hazard evaluation process. Adapted from Cairns [6].

system, testing should emphasize probable effects in aquatic model ecosystems. On the other hand, if the material will be released in a terrestrial system (e.g., an agricultural pesticide), testing should emphasize effects in model terrestrial systems. It must be remembered, however, that interconnections among ecosystems may allow materials to be transported from the site of release. A serious problem currently exists with nonpoint source pollution originating as runoff from urban streets, agricultural fields, and livestock areas. Although application of fertilizers and pesticides on farmlands generally produces desired effects, the effects become undesirable when the material is transferred to streams and rivers.

The second use for ecological assessment is in determining if an ecological effect has occurred after a release of potentially dangerous materials. In this regard, ecologists must understand the nature of the released material (i.e., the organism or its products), the expected fate and rate of transport of the material, the site of the release, and any other known secondary effects such as specific pathogenicity or genetic transfer. A summary of the nature of the information that can be obtained from different types of testing strategies is shown in Table 5.1.

Pathology

The public generally associates the generic term *bacteria* with organisms that cause disease. Additionally, a number of organisms under study for genetic manipulation have known pathogenic parent strains [18]. It is not possible to test a complete array of species that might be affected by novel,

Table 5.1. Summary of Potential Impacts and Assessment Methods for
Evaluating Ecological Effects of Genetically Altered Organisms

Impact	Methods	Parameters examined
Pathological	Histology	Tissue lesions
Toxicological: important and sensitive species	Dose-response	Mortality Growth Reproduction
Model ecosystem	Dose-response	Community structure (species number, diversity) Population dynamics Primary production Respiration Nutrient cycling
Ecosystem structure	Microcosm analysis Mesocosm analysis Field test Ecosystem survey	Population dynamics Population structure Community structure (species number, diversity) Biomass of selected groups or compartments
Ecosystem function	Microcosm analysis Mesocosm analysis Field test Ecosystem survey	Nutrient retention Nutrient cycling Detritus processing Respiration Primary production

introduced organisms. Nevertheless, laboratory screening procedures are necessary as one step in the regulatory process to estimate the probable pathogenicity of engineered organisms. Possible transformations of non-pathogenic strains after environmental exposure are unlikely, but also should be considered. In either case, environmental assessment probably will occur after release has occurred, and pathogenicity will not be detected until after widespread loss of a relatively narrow range of species. In many species, pathogenicity can only be detected by obvious body lesions that may be examined histologically [24] among larger species whose biology is well known. Pathological effects on microbial species probably will be detected only in model ecosystem experiments, as changes in community structure or system function. It might be argued that many species have the potential to mount an immunological response to a new pathogen. This ability is comparatively restricted, and it is probable that microorganisms and other organisms with rapid productive rates are more likely to have a population genetic response (i.e., survival of resistant types). A comparable response is unlikely in a larger species, since the generation time is too long to achieve appreciable genetic resistance to a new pathogen. The loss of the American chestnut because of an introduced fungal pathogen is a good example of this point.

Toxicology Paradigm

The release of novel microorganisms into the environment may be studied in a manner similar to that used to assess ecological impacts of toxic materials. The major difference between toxic materials and genetically engineered microorganisms is the potential ability of the latter to survive and increase in concentration through reproduction, and to mutate or hybridize with other organisms. Because of these inherent abilities, studies of transport and fate and of the genetic stability of genetically altered microorganisms in natural ecosystems are especially important. A toxic material released into a stream or river will generally decrease in concentration as distance from the source increases. Moreover, toxic chemicals, though they may persist in sediments or be concentrated through the food chain, are unlikely to move upstream or into neighboring ecosystems in significant concentrations. Released genetically altered microorganisms, however, may easily be transferred from one system to another and, if they survive, have an adverse impact. It is well known, for example, that migratory water-algae fowl are the source of transport for many influenza viruses. If an ecological assessment is to be made, it is especially important to be able to determine quickly and accurately the dose at any given site. This dose measurement can then be compared to known effects from model ecosystem experiments.

For biological materials that produce toxic chemicals, certain standard toxicity testing procedures are available to evaluate potential adverse effects on nontarget species [1]. These tests follow the typical pattern of dose-response testing using mortality, growth, and reproduction as end points. Additional tests are available for assessing toxicity rapidly and sensitively, but these rely on nontraditional end points [12,20] based on the behavior of model systems. In general, model systems, or microcosms, are used to evaluate effects of some perturbation on an ecological process that cannot be obtained in studies of single species. Such testing systems, for example, can be used to evaluate effects on nutrient cycling and carbon processing. These processes require the presence of a complex portion of a natural community and cannot be evaluated using traditional toxicological end points, although dose-response relationships can often be examined in model systems.

Microcosm tests can provide a great deal of valuable information in assessing the potential hazard of the release of novel organisms. They already have been used to examine survivorship of parental types in simulated nonnative habitats [18]. Additionally, microcosms should be useful in evaluating effects on ecologically important phenomena, such as nutrient cycling rates using sediment-water cores [3]. Such testing systems can evaluate the probability of adverse interactions in important detrital processing pathways by examining effects on nutrient regeneration and organic carbon mineralization. A variety of methods is available to follow community-level phenomena such as heterotrophic substrate utilization [9].

Adequate evaluation of potential adverse effects of novel organisms requires an understanding of their fate and persistence in differing life zones, that is, knowledge of where the organisms go after release and whether they continue to increase in number. These questions have been addressed succinctly by Rissler [25] (see Table 5.2). In general, evaluations of this sort need to be made on a site-specific or case-by-case basis [5].

Ecosystem Structural Analysis

Any ecosystem assessment must have a point of reference for comparing results. The simplest and most direct point of reference is a baseline of information regarding system structure before any impact occurs [13]. In this way a before-and-after comparison can be made, although the parameters measured (e.g., population sizes of particular species) may be confounded by seasonal fluctuations or by interactions with other populations in the system. A sufficient baseline of information is not available on most ecosystems over a variety of seasons and years to use as a point of reference.

An alternative approach to assessing before-and-after effects is the conventional control site method. One or more reference stations isolated from the impact in the ecosystem of interest are compared to a series of stations that supposedly were affected. Control sites ideally receive no impact. Depending on the fate of released genetically altered organisms, establishment of control sites within the ecosystem under study may be a substantial problem. The advantage of the control site method is that seasonal fluctuations and population responses that occur in cycles may be similar for a variety of sites within the same ecosystem, thus making comparisons among sites feasible.

Structural analyses of ecosystems generally require a large field team with expertise in sampling a variety of organisms at a number of stations, including the control and impacted stations. For a complete taxonomic survey of a given ecosystem, it might be necessary to sample active taxa ranging from microorganisms through the most complex species. This feat would be gargantuan if care were not taken to ensure that released genetically altered organisms sampled at one site were not transported by the researchers themselves to another site. The basic analytical technique is to assess numbers of species and population sizes (at least for the dominant species) in

Table 5.2. General Questions Proposed for Research on Biotic Environmental Effects of Deliberately Released Genetically Engineered Microorganisms

Event	Questions*
Contact with species or biological systems that the microorganisms can injure	What species or biological systems are exposed to the microorganisms?
	Is knowledge of the exposures associated with the unaltered parent organisms sufficient to predict the exposures of the engineered organisms?
	Do the intended pattern of use and knowledge of means of transport predict the species or systems to be exposed?
	What are the magnitude, frequency, duration, and routes of exposure?
	Are existing exposure assessment methodologies for microorganisms satisfactory for GEMs?
	Can engineered genes or other genes be transferred in nature to other organisms? Which ones?
	Can genes from other organisms be transferred to GEMs more readily than to naturally occurring ones? Why?

From Rissler [25], with permission.

*Delineated according to series of events leading to harm.

a variety of taxonomic groups and to compare these among stations. A well designed structural survey includes sampling at several different times or, if an acute impact is hypothesized, following populations at several sites over more than two or three generations.

Determination of adverse ecological effects is a statistical problem of detecting differences. Many parameters and indices have been used [13,17]. These can be summarized as significant population differences in response to stress, and as community differences in species density, richness, or diversity. If rigorous hypotheses are framed before field sampling is undertaken and sampling is planned to detect differences of a known magnitude among sites, it is comparatively simple to test statistical hypotheses of differences between impacted and unimpacted sites or in the same sites before and after a hypothesized stress [27].

Ecosystem Functional Analysis

Analysis of functional responses in ecosystems to supposed impacts follows the same general plan as for structural analysis. That is, a number of sampling sites in the ecosystem must be established, some in affected areas and others in areas supposedly receiving little or no disturbance. It is not possible to sample for a functional response rapidly. However, information can be collected on system function, including feeding, egestion, respiration, and primary production rates, using organisms or water samples. Furthermore, it is possible to remove and maintain sediment materials in the laboratory or to remove repeated samples over time to determine the rate of processing of carbon and inorganic nutrients [9].

Although broad boundaries have been drawn for the various processing rates of ecosystems, considerations of season and the relative state of the system based on previous history must be known, and results from functional analyses interpreted with caution, if environmental effects are to be inferred. Nevertheless, analyses of differences in processing rates among sites can be done using common statistical techniques, provided an estimate of the difference to be analyzed can be obtained. The processing of carbon and inorganic nutrients (N, P, S) is absolutely critical to the maintenance of system function. The range within which processing rates can vary and be considered acceptable also must be determined.

Nonspecies Effects

Genetically altered organisms may have a number of effects on the physical environment that are not directly measurable as effects on other organisms [30]. Since most bacteria, like other organisms, require living space on a natural substrate, it is likely that proliferation of novel or nonindigenous organisms could have substantial deleterious effects on natural and man-made formations. This problem is common in any ecosystem where a man-made device has been placed, and marine ecologists commonly refer to it as biofouling [32]. The accumulation of organisms on surfaces of any sort may preclude the invasion of other species and also render the colonized surface unusable, such as the drag resulting from the accumulation of barnacles on ship hulls. In addition to effects similar to fouling by naturally occurring species, genetically altered organisms may cause other types of damage. For example, they may produce and release corrosive materials that degrade metal or wooden structures. Films, scums, or floating mats of organisms with little ecological impact could easily clog intake filters or pipes for industries. Similarly, growth of these organisms on exchange surfaces, such as the pipes in commercial electric generation facilities, could reduce the efficiency of these installations, similar to the problem of intake pipe colonization by *Corbicula* [8a].

Growth of introduced organisms may have additional effects on the aesthetic value of the landscape. This effect can be caused by growth of organisms on major natural formations or man-made structures. Although there may be no immediate environmental impact, one must only think back to the dense growths of Kudzu along the east coast of the United States to be reminded of how unappealing seemingly uncontrolled single-species growth can be.

The propensity of introduced novel organisms to affect nonbiological components adversely could be examined concurrently with microcosm tests. For example, an array of possible substrates (concrete, steel, glass) could be added to microcosms and examined after several intervals of exposure to determine if corrosion or other effects had occurred. It is comparatively simple to examine materials using electron-scan microscopy and to quantify changes in introduced substrates. Anecdotal evidence from experiments provides additional information on unusual effects on man-made materials.

EVALUATION OF TEST METHODS
Lessons from Toxicology

The toxicological paradigm of dose-response relationships can provide a measure of the probability of adverse effects from the release of a particular novel organism under particular conditions. Applying toxicological methods to ecosystem protection, however, has been criticized as overly simplistic [19]. For example, arrays of single-species tests may have little relevance to predictions of effects on ecosystems. Ecosystems are not simply collections of species; they are complex interacting systems with emergent properties, and are greater than the sum of their parts [14,29]. Therefore, predictive testing must account for important characteristics of the potential receiving ecosystem if test results are to be directly applied to estimating hazard. Conversely, delineation of the ecosystem properties to be protected should suggest the type of testing system needed. In general, microcosm testing systems that retain many features of the portion of the system likely to be affected should serve as the basis for ecological effect evaluations. Simultaneous evaluation of several potential effects (e.g., pathogenicity, ecological process, or nonspecies effects) of novel organisms is then possible, rather than relying on a tiered testing program that takes longer to achieve results [7].

To determine the probability of adverse effects occurring as a result of a planned or unplanned release of genetically altered organisms, response thresholds must be measured directly as part of the hazard evaluation process. There is considerable evidence that microcosm and mesocosm testing systems are sufficiently environmentally realistic to allow ecologists to measure the necessary response levels directly [12]. The current regulatory strategy that compiles large amounts of data generated without a predetermined plan is scientifically unjustifiable. The data base for most toxic chemicals is compiled, and then various correction factors are applied to the data, depending on the nature of the test (e.g., duration, rate of toxicant replacement, verification of toxicant concentration). The relative contribution of ameliorating factors also is taken into account, and an extrapolation is made to a supposedly acceptable effect level (i.e., roughly protecting 95% of the resident species in the receiving system). Developing a sufficient data base to make such an estimation requires a minimum of about 18 months and may take several years. This is especially burdensome to industries developing new materials and may be unnecessary, since it is probably not possible to test an adequate array of species for all the potential receiving ecosystems. An alternative to this procedure has been the testing of many species simultaneously in some form of model ecosystem. If a model ecosystem has a sufficient number of characteristics of the more complex system it was designed to simulate, estimates of effect can be based directly on the behavior of the model ecosystem and do not necessarily rely on extrapolation of data generated unsystematically. Coincidentally, recent evidence indicates that estimated effect levels for microecosystems correspond closely to criteria estimated from large data bases of single-species tests. If this is the case, and ecologists agree upon the adequacy of the complex testing system employed, testing a large array of species individually is unnecessary to determine those species that are resistant or sensitive to introduced materials. The same information can be obtained more quickly and at a substantially lower cost from microecosystem tests.

The most difficult problem with interpreting microecosystem test results is the diversity of testing systems used. These test systems will not provide an acceptable alternative to the simpler, direct toxicity tests currently in use until ecologists agree upon the salient characteristics that should be included in the test systems and upon the important parameters that should be measured in response to disturbances. If some model ecosystems could be agreed upon as standard tests, and a similar number of reference ecosystems were used for initial validation and calibration, testing a large array of possible environmental disturbances should be reasonably simple.

Ecosystem Assessment

Determination of adverse ecological effects assumes that either a sufficiently detailed pretreatment data base exists (and is relevant) or that unaffected control areas can be designated for comparison purposes.

Although evaluating ecological impacts on either basis is statistically questionable [17], there remains little alternative to such site-specific studies. A sufficient data base is not presently available so that the expectations for species occurrence patterns or material processing rates can be stated a priori, except in the most general terms. General or order-of-magnitude estimates are insufficient to detect differences between affected and unaffected areas.

Structural analysis of ecosystems has not changed a great deal over the last 40 years. It is still necessary to collect a large amount of data, including biological and environmental samples (e.g., water, sediment, soil), for determination of the background variability in the system and for inclusion in the analysis of factors that might contribute to large or small population sizes of important species. The state-of-the-art procedures for structural analysis have commonly been called "critter counting," with the implication that this is an inferior sort of biological sampling. In reality, organisms in their natural habitats affected by introduced materials integrate the effects of any disturbance. The problem with critter counting has been that a huge, complex mass of data is generated over a relatively short period of time, and professionals sifting through this information usually end up confused, resulting in a focus on simplified portions of data that are then used to infer environmental health or damage.

It is no longer necessary to be overwhelmed by massive, complex data sets. Use of high-speed computers with large capacities to process information has resulted in the development of statistical procedures that can reduce these data sets [11,16]. These procedures generally involve the creation of synthetic, composite variables; for example, the large amount of water quality information commonly produced by repeated sampling of study sites may be reduced to two or three composite factors. Comparisons can then be made among these composite variables, based on the occurrence and numbers of individuals of the various taxa collected at the study sites. The most significant drawback to higher-level statistical analysis is the lack of agreement in interpretation. In addition, communicating the results of an analytical procedure to audiences not familiar with such techniques may be difficult.

Functional analyses of ecosystems may reduce the number of variables measured by examining a limited array of possible responses. In some respects these analyses reduce the complexity of the system so that certain fundamental properties are examined. The analysis of the information (i.e., detecting differences among stations or study sites) may be simpler, since the data set is arbitrarily limited by the factors studied. For impacts of genetically altered organisms that might be felt at the detritus-bacteria level of the ecosystem, these sorts of analyses may be especially appropriate

[9,21]. Examination of higher groups, especially those that depend on the bacteria-detritus pool for food and inorganic nutrients, may be an equally viable alternative. Studies of functional processes have the same sampling and seasonal difficulties experienced with taxonomic units. As noted elsewhere in this chapter, it is possible for functional responses to remain the same, despite adverse effects on resident species. That is, some species may be stimulated and others adversely affected, resulting in no appreciable change in system function. To the systems ecologist, if system function remains the same, no adverse impact has taken place. To a more traditional, organism-centered ecologist, a radical shift in population size or structure or in community composition directly related to a measured dose of foreign material would be interpreted as an adverse effect.

In addition to evaluating effects on important processes, it is necessary to evaluate the innate variability of systems likely to be affected by engineering organisms. For temperate ecosystems, the range of variability in processing rates is thought to be closely related to annual seasonal variability. The range of variability may not be similar for geographically proximate and otherwise similar systems. In studies of reclaimed lakes in central Florida, for example, Boody et al. [2] found extensive variability in ecosystems of similar histories, basin morphologies, and trophic status. Although seasonal patterns were evident in primary production, there was broad variation in the timing and magnitude of seasonal maxima and minima.

Gaps in Ecological Data

At the present time, no general agreement has been reached among ecologists as to what parameters should be measured to assess adverse ecological effects. There are compelling arguments on both sides of the structure/function argument. Ecologists have studied a comparatively narrow range of available ecosystems, using many different techniques. There are no standard methods in the engineering sense of the term, although certain measurements routinely are taken in certain ways. The standardization of measurement techniques basically has followed the technological development of measuring instruments. This development has been generally beneficial to ecologists, since the technological development of measuring instruments has allowed environmental measures to become more precise. Adequate information is still not available, however, upon which to make a priori predictions of population sizes for keystone species or narrow-range predictions of processing rates for particular compounds. Failing this information, ecological assessment studies depend upon the use of in-system control areas and suffer from replication problems. Regulatory agencies must realize that the current extent of knowledge about ecosystems is still comparatively sparse, even though a large number of studies have been undertaken.

The basic problem with using existing data as a baseline is that it is frequently impossible to use exactly the same methods, either because the methods are incorrect and the data are therefore suspect, or because we have modest abilities to repeat the judgments made by the original investigators. It would be useful if a systematic survey of ecosystems, similar to the river surveys conducted by the Academy of Natural Sciences (Philadelphia), were resumed with the purpose of fingerprinting some of the major ecosystems, using the same methodological approach in all the systems studied.

Ecological End Points

The determination of an end point to measure environmental stress is not likely to be satisfactory for those who wish a single, all-purpose "generic" end point suitable for all regions and climates and easily used by people with various degrees of training. As Slobodkin [26] notes:

> In contrast to molecular genetics and biochemistry, which have at times had a relatively small number of empirical questions that needed answering before understanding could advance, central focal questions do not generally exist in ecology. There are no single obvious-next-questions. The problems of ecology span the full range of interactions among the earth's two million species of organisms and their environment. Production of a unitary, comprehensible, ecological theory is thus completely intractable. There is no present hope for deriving the mechanistic basis of, say, a tropical rain forest in the same way that one can begin to understand the mechanistic basis for nerve conduction, muscle contraction, or photosynthesis.

The response thresholds (i.e., the concentration of material below which no observable effects occur) will be different for different species, for different life history stages within a species, and with different levels of biological organization (i.e., population, community, or ecosystem). Therefore, the question is: What characteristics of a particular ecosystem are to be protected? Presumably there are a number of characteristics of both ecological and social importance. In some cases, one or two end points may be selected, either because they are more sensitive or because they are so closely linked to other attributes of the biological system that it is impossible to affect one without affecting the other. In other words, considerable information redundancy occurs, and collecting the same information in different ways is not cost effective. There is no way to protect complex and regionally different ecosystems without a skilled site-specific analysis. Unfortunately, laws and regulations often are written in such a way that they obstruct scientifically justifiable efforts to solve even the most obvious problems in simple, cost-effective ways. Instead of focusing on the desired end point and attempting to reason together to achieve a particular goal, the regulated and the regulators are forced into a contentious, noncooperative relationship. Ecologists in other countries — particularly those in Canada, who are in a good position to observe our actions closely — are astounded at the degree to which legal requirements dominate scientific judgment. There ideally should be no prescriptive list of end points or effects, but only general guidelines, with perhaps illustrative case histories of solutions of problems in particular ecosystems. Fortunately, such case histories abound in the literature. A few situations will serve to illustrate the relationship between end point and environmental management goals.

Protection of an Endangered Species of Fish. Among the many changes that are characteristic of ecosystems is replacement of species with other species in a succession process well recognized by ecologists the world over. However, if the management goal is to protect a rare or endangered species, conditions most suitable to the preservation of that species must be maintained, even if interference with normal ecosystem change is involved. For example, if the species requires a certain type of substrate for spawning that is being made unsuitable because of imperfect natural invasion of a plant species, the plant species should be removed. End points in this particular case are at the species level and include growth, reproductive success, recruitment rate, and the like. Other normally important end points, such as detritus processing, energy flow, trophic structural relationships, and species richness, are secondary and are important only in terms of protecting a particular species.

Preservation of a Wilderness Area. In attempting to preserve a forest, "wild river," or some other ecosystem that the nature conservancy considers particularly important, management goals would focus on community or ecosystem-level characteristics. These are at a higher level of biological organization than single species, and the end points should reflect this feature. Suitable end points might include the detritus-processing rates for a headwater stream, or nutrient and energy flow for a forest ecosystem, including watershed and perhaps trophic-level relationships within the community.

Preservation of a Perturbation-Dependent Ecosystem. This type of ecosystem [28] becomes ecologically senescent if it is not perturbed (i.e., disturbed) periodically, as illustrated in Figure 5.3. A good example of a perturbation-dependent ecosystem is one that is fire-dependent, such as the New Jersey pine barrens, prairie grasslands, or the Great Basin

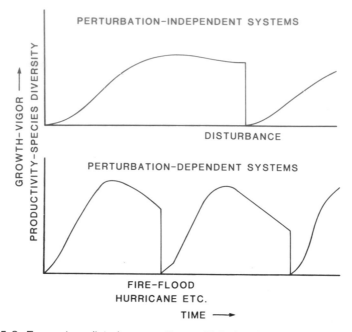

Figure 5.3. Ecosystem disturbance patterns. Disturbances in general ecosystems create vegetational setbacks and complete recovery is slow, whereas disturbances in perturbation-dependent ecosystems usually stimulate pulses of growth that rapidly decline unless disturbed again. From Vogl [28].

shrub-steppe. Flood-plain ecosystems undergo periodic disturbance through flooding to maintain ecological vigor. End points differ depending on the ecological stage of the system, that is, disturbance, immediate postdisturbance, intermediate recovery, or full recovery. It is a sine qua non that one must not only know something about the end points characteristic of the present stage, but also something about the succeeding stages. Therefore, a time series or spectral statistical analysis would be appropriate, and the end points should be selected accordingly.

A Perturbation-Independent Ecosystem. These ecosystems, ranging from coral reefs to tropical rain forests, are characterized by enormous richness of species and are relatively stable in their system-level attributes, such as nutrient and energy cycling.

End points for monitoring or accessing such systems could include species diversity, nutrient cycling, trophic relationships, and perhaps predator–prey relationships, and key or controlling species, among others.

This illustrative material is intended to show how different end points may be used to achieve quality-control objectives in different ecosystems and biological situations. Even within each of these categories, the end points might differ considerably among ecosystems and geographic regions. There are enormous differences, for example, in areas with high and low rainfall or marked temperature stability. In selecting end points one must be certain that the information to be generated is useful in terms of the decision under consideration and the type of system being assessed. On a *CBS Today* news broadcast, there was mention of the Supreme Court decision by Justice White that nationwide standards for environmental protection should be viewed with flexibility for a particular regional decision. Presumably, such flexibility includes both the selection of end points and the determination of the appropriate thresholds of concern for the region.

CONCLUSIONS

Failing a groundswell of public opinion, support, and funding, ecological assessments have an important place in the regulation of the release of genetically altered organisms. If a careful series of tests is conducted to establish potential ecological effects of these novel organisms, then it should be obvious, based on the results of these tests, which ecological parameters are most important to measure in the "real world." Table 5.3 summarizes attributes that require assessment and shows how differing organisms may be ranked for potential effect. The testing system should include microcosm tests that examine potential effects on key components of ecosystems, followed by more elaborate field tests in which measurements are taken of effects on potentially sensitive taxa and processes based on the results of the

Table 5.3. Attributes of Introduced Organisms of Potential Importance in Ecological Assessment*

Attribute
Transportability of disemules
Colonization potential
Persistence
Partitioning — critical compartment
Transfer of genetic material to other organisms
Potential of seasonal dominance
Probable recovery of ecosystem if displaced in structure or function

*By rating available knowledge about each attribute, a relative score can be obtained to rank organisms.

microcosm tests. Assuming that a material is deemed safe for use in the environment or is licensed to be discharged into the environment at a given rate, ecological assessments should be planned to validate predictions from microcosm and field trials. Such assessments should focus on expected critical taxa and processes, but also make some evaluation of the general state of biota and other processes not expected to be affected. An ecological assessment of this sort, which includes both structural and functional measurements, has the advantage of directing most of its energy at critical areas in making spot checks on the health of supposedly unaffected taxa and functions. Evaluation of nontarget processes and species could be used in support of contentions that the introduced material has little or no adverse effect. This support is only qualitative, however, since it continues to be difficult to validate a null prediction.

The greatest need at the present time is not for the development of new ecological assessment tools for use in natural ecosystems, but rather the development of adequate predictive tools, including predictive models, that estimate effects based on controlled laboratory or field enclosure studies. By devising direct, simple measures of ecological function and by adequately assessing these in field trials, it will become obvious which parameters need to be measured to determine if adverse ecological effects have occurred. It seems clear that effects of introduced microorganisms are likely to be noted in displacement of natural microbial populations, interference with the functioning of native microbial communities, or the passage of genetic material from introduced organisms to native species. The greatest potential appears to be for interference with normal biogeochemical processes. Additionally, interaction of microbial populations may result in alteration of the host range for pathogenic or opportunistic species.

The greatest weakness of the current application of existing methods to ecological assessments is usually the inadequacy of sample size. That is, an insufficient number of replicate measurements are taken at any given study site. This is perplexing but understandable, since the amount of time required to process samples of organisms or to conduct meaningful trials examining system function can be extraordinarily large. The end result is that ecological studies conducted over a large portion of an ecosystem become extraordinarily expensive. Consequently, it is even more important to develop standard methods for assessing ecologically important parameters than has been the case in the past. Scientists have expressed a genuine fear that genetically engineered organisms might perform in unpredictable ways. Experience has shown that these initial fears are somewhat overstated [4]. Since the application of genetically engineered organisms in the environment has been limited to small-scale field trials, it is too early to evaluate the fears of ecologists that widespread alteration of nutrient cycles or structural aspects of ecosystems will take place, based on the release of these organisms. Nevertheless, no one has a desire to be careless in allowing one more disturbance to affect ecosystems already disturbed to some degree by human activities.

REFERENCES

1. American Society for Testing and Materials. 1980. Conducting acute toxicity tests with fishes, macroinvertebrates, and amphibians. In *Annual Book of ASTM Standards.* American Society for Testing and Materials, Philadelphia, pp. 282-308.
2. Boody, O. C., C. D. Pollman, G. H. Tourtelotte, R. E. Dickinson, and A. N. Arcuri. 1984. *Ecological Considerations of Reclaimed Lakes in Central Florida's Phosphate Region.* Florida Institute of Phosphate Research, Bartow, Fla.
3. Bourquin, A. W., R. L. Garnas, P. H. Pritchard, F. G. Wilkes, C. R. Cripe, and N. I. Rubinstein. 1979. Interdependent microcosms for the assessment of pollutants in the marine environment. *Int. J. Environ. Stud. 13*:131-140.
4. Brill, W. J. 1985. Safety concerns and genetic engineering in agriculture. *Science 227*:381-384.
5. Brown, J. H., R. K. Colwell, R. E. Leuski, B. R. Levin, M. Cloyd, P. J. Regal, and D. S. Simberloff. 1984. Report on workshop on possible ecological and evolutionary impacts of bioengineered organisms released into the environment. *Bull. Ecol. Soc. America 65*:436-438.
6. Cairns, J., Jr. 1980. Estimating hazard. *BioScience 30*:101-107.
7. Cairns, J., Jr. 1983. The case for simultaneous toxicity testing at different levels of biological organization. In W. E. Bishop, R. D. Cardwell, and B. B. Heidolph (Eds.), *Aquatic Toxicology and Hazard Assessment: Sixth Symposium.* American Society for Testing and Materials, Philadelphia, pp. 111-127.
8. Chakrabarty, A. M., J. S. Karns, J. J. Kilbane, and D. K. Chatterjee. 1984. Selective evolution of genes for enhanced degradation of persistent, toxic chemicals. In W. Arber, K. Illmanssee, W. J. Peacock, and P. Starlinger (Eds.), *Genetic Manipulation: Impact on Man and Society.* International Council of Scientific Union Press, Cambridge, England, pp. 43-54.
8a. Cairns, J., Jr. and D. S. Cherry. 1983. A site-specific field and laboratory evaluation of fish and asiatic clam population responses to coal-fired power plant discharges. *Water Sci. Techn. 15*:31-58.
9. Costerton, J. W. and R. R. Colwell, Eds. 1979. *Native Aquatic Bacteria: Enumeration, Activity, and Ecology.* American Society for Testing and Materials, Philadelphia, pp. 1-214.
10. Fenchel, T. and T. H. Blackburn. 1979. *Bacteria and Mineral Cycling.* Academic Press, New York.
11. Gauch, H. G. 1977. ORDIFLEX — a flexible computer program for four ordination techniques. Ecology and Systematics, Cornell University, Ithaca, N.Y.
12. Giesy, J., Ed. 1980. *Microcosms in Ecological Research.* Conference 78101. National Technical Information Service, Springfield, Va.
13. Green, R. H. 1979. *Sampling Design and Statistical Methods for Environmental Biologists.* John Wiley and Sons, New York.
14. Heath, R. G., J. W. Spann, and J. F. Freitzer. 1969. Marked DDE impairment of mallard reproduction in controlled studies. *Nature 224*:47-48.

15. Hellawell, J. M. 1978. *Biological Surveillance of Rivers*. Water Research Centre, Stevenage, England.
16. Hill, M. O. 1979. DECORANA — a FORTRAN program for detrended correspondence analysis and reciprocal averaging. Ecology and Systematics, Cornell University, Ithaca, N.Y.
17. Hurlbert, S. H. 1984. Pseudoreplication and the design of ecological field experiments. *Ecol. Monogr. 54*:187–211.
18. Liang, L. N., J. L. Sinclair, L. M. Mallory, and M. Alexander. 1982. Fate in model ecosystems of microbial species of potential use in genetic engineering. *Appl. Environ. Microsc. 44*:708–714.
19. National Academy of Sciences. 1980. *Testing for the Effects of Chemicals on Ecosystems*. National Academy Press, Washington, DC.
20. Niederlehner, B. R., J. R. Pratt, A. L. Buikema, Jr., and J. Cairns, Jr. 1985. Laboratory tets evaluating the effects of cadmium on freshwater protozoan communities. *Environ. Toxicol. Chem. 4*:155–165.
21. Nisbitt, B. 1984. *Nutrition and Feeding Strategies in Protozoa*. Croom Helm, London.
22. Odum, H. T. 1983. *Systems Ecology*. John Wiley and Sons, New York.
23. Poole, R. W. 1974. *An Introduction to Quantitative Ecology*. McGraw-Hill, New York.
24. Post, G. W. 1983. *Textbook of Fish Health*. TFH Publications, Neptune City, N.J.
25. Rissler, J. F. 1984. Research needs for biotic environmental effects of genetically engineered organisms. *Recombinant DNA Tech. Bull. 7*:20–30.
26. Slobodkin, L. B. 1984. Toward a global perspective. *BioScience 34*:484–485.
27. Sokal, R. R. and F. J. Rohlf. 1983. *Biometry*. W. H. Freeman, San Francisco, Cal.
28. Vogl, R. J. 1980. The ecological factors that produce perturbation-dependent ecosystems. In J. Cairns, Jr. (Ed.), *The Recovery Process in Damaged Ecosystems*. Ann Arbor Science Publishers, Ann Arbor, Mich., pp. 63–94.
29. Webster, J. R. 1979. Hierarchical organization of ecosystems. In A. Halfon (Ed.), *Theoretical Systems Ecology*. Academic Press, New York, pp. 119–129.
30. Westman, W. E. 1985. *Ecology, Impact Assessment and Environmental Planning*. John Wiley and Sons, New York.
31. Wetzel, R. G. 1983. *Limnology*. 2nd ed. W. B. Saunders, Philadelphia.
32. Woods Hole Oceanographic Institution. 1952. *Marine Fouling and Its Prevention*. U.S. Naval Institute, Washington, D.C.

6

Assessing the Transport and Fate of Bioengineered Microorganisms in the Environment

Lawrence W. Barnthouse and Anthony V. Palumbo

The risk that a bioengineered microorganism deliberately released into the environment will have unanticipated adverse health and environmental effects is a function of its ability to proliferate in the environment in which it is released, its rate or probability of transport to other environments, its ability to establish and proliferate in the new environment, and its effects on the invaded environment. This chapter specifically deals with the problem of environmental transport and fate.

Given that the microbe in question can survive and proliferate in the environment in which it is released, how likely is it to disperse away from the release site? How far and how rapidly will the transported microbes move? Can they survive long enough to reach target environments or hosts? To answer these questions, it is necessary to identify the various pathways through which microorganisms can move; quantify their dispersal rates along these pathways; and to estimate their survival rates in air, water, and soil.

In this chapter we review the methods currently available for quantifying the transport and fate of microbes in atmospheric and aqueous media and assess their adequacy for purposes of risk assessment. We review the literature on transport and fate of microorganisms, including studies of pathways of migration, the survival of microorganisms during transport, and methods that have been used to model microbial transport and fate. In addition, we review the transport and fate models that have been used in environmental risk assessments for radionuclides and toxic chemicals and evaluate their applicability to the problem of assessing environmental risks of bioengineered microorganisms.

This chapter is strictly concerned with the transport of microorganisms between patches of favorable environment separated by unfavorable patches within which growth and reproduction are not possible (e.g., corn-fields separated by forest). Phenomena occurring within favorable patches, such as proliferation and plasmid exchange, are outside the scope of this review. In addition, it should be recognized that the overall risk assessment process for bioengineered organisms will probably resemble the process employed in assessing other forms of risk. Both generic assessments of tech-nologies and site-specific assessments of particular applications may be per-formed; hence, no single model will be adequate for all assessments. As has been the case for other environmental stresses, limits on time, resources, and scientific understanding will make it impossible to develop highly accu-rate numerical risk assessments based on models that faithfully reproduce every process that influences the fate and transport of microbes. The avail-ability, accuracy, and precision of data are as important in choices of mod-els as is mechanistic realism [5].

OVERVIEW OF INFORMATION ON THE TRANSPORT
AND FATE OF MICROORGANISMS
IN THE ENVIRONMENT

Key factors in the transport of microorganisms in the environment include the size of the source population, the rate of dispersal of organisms along environmental pathways, and the survival of the organisms during transport. The size of the source population and the ability of the organ-isms to survive during transport will differ depending on the type of organ-isms released. Inadvertent or accidental release of genetically engineered microorganisms will probably involve small source populations. Microor-ganisms engineered to produce pharmaceuticals or industrial chemicals will be grown under controlled conditions and can be altered or weakened to minimize their chances of survival following accidental release. However, microorganisms designed for use in agriculture or pollution control may well be altered to increase their rate of survival and growth in the environ-ment. They may be released in large numbers and be transported in a via-ble state over long distances.

There are three major pathways for the transport of microorganisms in the environment. These include transmission by air, by water, and by ani-mal or technological vectors. The dispersal of pathogenic microorganisms has been assumed to be dominated by one pathway, usually direct contact

[58], but it recently has become evident that multiple dispersal modes are common [15,58]. It is likely that multiple dispersal modes are also important in the transport of nonpathogenic microorganisms. Disease transmission by direct contact between infected and uninfected hosts, though the dominant dispersal pathway for many pathogens, is outside the scope of this chapter.

Aerial Dispersal

Airborne microorganisms can originate from both human and nonhuman sources. Bacteria are injected into the atmosphere by human activities that produce dust (e.g., vehicle operation, manufacturing, and construction) and from sources such as solid waste and sewage treatment plants [63]. Microorganisms in water can become airborne through wave action or bubble bursting, and microorganisms on soil or vegetation can be transported into the atmosphere through wind or thermal convection.

Because of their small size, bacteria and viruses settle out of the atmosphere at slow rates and can effectively be transported over long distances. For example, at a wind speed of 5 m/s, a 1 μm and a 5 μm bacterium would be transported 170 and 7 km, respectively, and settle at 1 m [14]. Bacteria are known to be transported in the atmosphere for hundreds to thousands of kilometers [13,14,104]. Virus particles could be transported even more effectively. Windborne viruses may have spread foot-and-mouth disease over 100 km of open sea to England from France [39].

Bacteria associated with aerosols or airborne soil particles settle more rapidly. Again assuming a wind speed of 5 m/s, a 10 μm and a 100 μm particle would be transported, respectively, 830 m and 12 m and settle at 1 m [45]. Association with particles, however, may facilitate the long-range transport of bacteria by increasing their rate of survival [2]. Bacteria are sensitive to drying, and large particles reach hygroscopic equilibrium more slowly than small particles.

Several approaches have been used to model the aerial dispersal of microorganisms. Gaussian plume dispersion models, modified to include bacterial death rates, have been used to predict dispersal gradients [62,81]. Plant disease dispersal gradients have been modeled with turbulent diffusion models [41] and with empirical models [40,41].

Waterborne Dispersal

Although many enteric diseases are caused by water-dispersed microorganisms [25,101], minimal data are available on dispersal gradients in water. The transport of microorganisms in surface water depends primarily on the movement of the water. However, the attachment of bacteria to particles greatly complicates the problem of modeling microbial transport in this medium. Microbe–particle association is much more complicated than the partitioning of chemical contaminants and is not amenable to modeling using simple partitioning coefficients. Bacteria use a variety of mechanisms to attach to surfaces [21]. Moreover, the ability to attach varies among bacterial species [83] and even with culture conditions [32]. Some bacteria undergoing starvation increase their hydrophobicity and thus increase their capacity to bind to solid surfaces [52].

The transport of microorganisms in ground water is strongly dependent on the interactions of microbes with the soil. Bacteria are filtered out by passing through the soil [36]; both bacteria and viruses are adsorbed to soil particles [37]. In unsaturated soil, bacteria may move only a few centimeters [43]. Much greater transport is possible in saturated soil [43,56], especially in coarse-textured or fractured strata [85].

Viable bacteria have been reported to move more than 900 m in ground water [35].

Animal Vectors

Animal vectors are highly effective dispersal mechanisms for many microorganisms. Maguire [66] found that algae, ciliates, flagellates, and moss spores are transported readily between water bodies by birds, insects, lizards, and racoons. Fish have been found to carry fecal coliform bacteria and streptococcus within their intestinal tracts for up to 14 days when those microorganisms are present in the water [34]. It is likely that other organisms capable of surviving in the intestinal tracts of fish are transported similarly. Plant bacterial diseases [23,88] and arboviruses [44,68] often are spread by insects. Bacterial attachment to copepods [48] or algae [78] could also be important in influencing bacterial transport in water.

Factors Affecting the Survival of Microorganisms during Transport

The relative importance of the factors influencing survival of microorganisms in the environment depends on the characteristics of both the environment and the organism. Bacteria that are resistant to starvation and abiotic stress and also have the ability to coexist with antagonistic species may best be able to survive introduction to a new environment [64].

Temperature is an important determinant of survival. In many studies, the effects of temperature and season are difficult to separate. In general, survival is decreased in the summer or at high temperatures [51,82,98]; however, there are exceptions [87]. In a study of the persistence of protozoan spores in soil Germida [38], it was theorized that longer persistence at low temperatures is related to decreased activity of the indigenous soil community. Thus, the slower die-off of fecal coliforms at low temperatures in sludge applied to soil [30] may be due to the effect of the sludge on the indigenous community. High temperatures may also reduce survival by increasing the likelihood of starvation due to accelerated metabolic demand.

Moisture can be important in determining survival of bacteria in soil [103] and air. Resistance of different bacterial strains and genera in soil to desiccation is highly variable [19,76,77,98]. Soil type also affects survival of introduced species [65,67,77]. The attachment of bacteria to particles may provide some protection to airborne bacteria from desiccation [2], and adsorption of bacteria to soil may increase their persistence [1].

The presence of other microorganisms may reduce the chance of survival of an introduced species. Survival of bacteria introduced in sterilized environments is often greater than survival in similar nonsterile environments [34,90]. The survival of bacteria in ground water may be better than in other aquatic systems where the total bacterial population is large. For example, *Shigella* added to wells could be recovered after 22 days, but survived only 30 minutes to 4 days in river water [34]. The relative absence of eukaryotic organisms in ground water may also increase chances for survival of bacteria, because protozoans that can reduce bacterial populations [42] are not present. Nutrients can affect the survival of introduced species. Many natural environments are nutrient-poor or have indigenous populations that can effectively outcompete introduced species for nutrients. Thus, resistance to starvation is often important to survival, and the addition of organic or inorganic nutrients can increase the chance of survival of introduced species [18,54]. However, the addition of nutrients can also decrease survival [18,53].

Physical and chemical factors such as light and pH can also influence bacterial survival. High light levels reduce bacterial survival in soils [98], in aerosols [29], and in water [86]. Survival of bacteria in water may be decreased by very low pH (4) [24,98] or very high pH (8 or 9) [73].

A wide range of survival times has been reported for bacteria in the environment. First-order die off rates for bacteria and viruses have been estimated by fitting data to an exponential decay model [10]. Estimated decay constants for bacteria in ground water range from 0.03 to 0.32 d-1 [36]. Higher mortality rates (e.g., 0.768 d-1 [9]) have been observed in seawater. Mortality of airborne bacteria is believed to be even higher. Based on literature data for laboratory cultures, bacterial death rates of 0.0001 to 0.01 s-1 (8.64 to 864 d-1) were used to model the fate of airborne bacteria [81].

Studies of the survival of bacteria in lake water and soil have shown that the data often fit a first-order exponential decay model for only the initial portion of an experiment. After a period of exponential decline, the number of bacteria often stabilizes [61,90]. Based on such observations, Alexander [1] has suggested that the survival of introduced bacteria follows several patterns. Some bacterial species show a rapid decline and are eliminated within 3 days; others show a logarithmic decline over 7 to 10 days, leaving a few remaining cells that persist much longer. Another pattern is a logarithmic decline for 1 to 14 days with little subsequent change in numbers.

All reported estimates of microbial mortality rates must be interpreted with caution. Much of the literature on the survival of microorganisms was written before it was known that bacteria can be "injured" so that they are not enumerated using standard techniques. It has been demonstrated that bacteria can become injured in drinking water, surface water, and wastewater [3,8,16,60,61,92]. Bacteria may survive in this state longer than indicated by some studies, and under some circumstances may again be able to grow and multiply. Hence, experimentally determined microbial mortality rates may often underestimate the abundance of viable microorganisms in the environment.

AVAILABLE MODELS FOR QUANTIFYING ENVIRONMENTAL TRANSPORT: PESTICIDES AND TOXIC CHEMICALS

In many respects, the processes governing the transport and fate of microbes resemble those of radionuclides, pesticides, and toxic chemicals. Like microbes, chemicals often are transported in association with aerosols, soil, and sediment particles. The movements of microbial particles are driven by the same physical forces that govern the transport of chemicals via air and water. As will be shown below, the transport of chemicals, like that of microbes, is complicated by sorption kinetics and intermedia transfer (e.g., settling and volatilization). The decay of radionuclides and the biochemical transformation of pesticides and toxic chemicals are similarly analogous to the death of microbes.

A great variety of models have been developed for use in assessing health and environmental risks of these substances. The same models, with minimal modification, often have been adapted to all three types of substances. They vary in spatial scale from meters to tens of kilometers and in temporal resolution from seconds to years. They have been developed for both generic and site-specific assessments, with vastly differing data requirements. In this section we briefly describe the purposes and characteristics of four types of models that appear relevant to biotechnology risk assessment: atmospheric transport and deposition, runoff, surface water, and ground water.

Atmospheric Transport
and Deposition Models

Models for predicting the fate of radionuclides and toxic chemicals in the atmosphere can be divided into two classes: near-field and far-field. Near-field models are intended for use within 50 km of the contaminant source. Although there are many computer codes for calculating near-field behavior of atmospheric pollutants, nearly all are variants of a single basic model, the Gaussian plume. In its simplest form, the Gaussian plume predicts the diffusion and dispersion of a conservative, gaseous plume from a continuous point source elevated above the ground, under constant wind speed and homogeneous atmospheric conditions, and over uniformly flat terrain. Many variations on the basic model have been developed to account for plume buoyancy, atmospheric stratification, wet and dry deposition of particles and aerosols, contaminant degradation or decay, ground-level and areal sources, and complex terrain.

Much of the model development and validation has been performed in connection with studies of radionuclide releases [47,93]. Several of the computer codes developed for radionuclide assessment subsequently have been modified for use with other pollutants. Two examples are ATM [84] and AIRDOS-EPA [71,96]. Both of these models compute ground-level atmospheric concentrations and deposition rates as functions of distance and direction from the pollutant source. Both account for decay or degradation, but neither accounts for complex terrain. Based on the validation studies that have been performed, it has been concluded [47] that Gaussian plume models can predict annual average atmospheric concentrations at distances of 10 km or less over relatively flat terrain with a factor of 2 accuracy. Predictions over time scales of a few hours or days are much less accurate.

A variety of non-Gaussian models have been developed for predicting far-field transport [46,72] and short-term near-field transport over complex terrain [57,97]. Although they extend the range of spatial and temporal scales that can be modeled, these codes are more demanding in terms of meteorological data requirements and are less flexible.

Runoff

The basic premise underlying the runoff models used in fate assessments of radionuclides and contaminants is that the surface transport of contaminants is driven primarily by rainfall, overland flow, and erosion. Consequently, the models are essentially of the rate of soil erosion as a function of rainfall, soil characteristics, slope, and vegetative cover. Properties of the contaminants themselves, such as solubility and degradability, are modeled as simple partition coefficients and first-order rate constants.

Mills et al. [69] described a screening-level approach to modeling contaminant deposition, runoff volume, and sediment erosion based on the universal soil loss equation [100]. The information required to employ their approach includes estimates of seven empirically determined factors describing rainfall, soil erodibility, slope, cover, and sediment delivery. Tables and figures for estimating these factors are provided in the report. The universal soil-loss equation originally was developed to estimate annual erosion potential. Because events on shorter time scales are important in determining rates of pollutant loading to surface water, a modified version developed by Williams [99] is used to model runoff and erosion during single storm events. The storm runoff model requires estimates of the runoff volume and peak runoff rate; methods for estimating both parameters are presented in the report [69].

While erosion is the basic force that moves substances deposited on the soil surface, substance-specific factors such as solubility, sorption, and degradation also affect rates of removal and delivery to surface water. Mills et al. [69] present modifications of the basic soil erosion model designed to account for the overland transport of nitrogen, phosphorus, and pesticides. The pesticide model includes both degradation and soil–water partitioning. Given estimates of pesticide application, pesticide disappearance (sum of first-order rates for volatilization and degradation), and octanol-water partitioning coefficient, the model calculates the total pesticide loss for a given storm event.

More complex models of runoff and erosion are available [6,22,27] in which the universal soil-loss equation and its empirically derived parameters are replaced by mechanistic descriptions of hydrological processes, such as interception, evapotranspiration, infiltration, percolation, and interflow. The hydrologic cycle is modeled in continuous time, using meteorological data defined on an hourly basis. Some of the models can follow multiple areas or catchments; for example, several fields containing different crops, or a field surrounded by forest. Provisions may be made for simulating the effects of erosion-control technologies on sediment and contaminant transport. Some of the most sophisticated models [49,75,80] link runoff models for multiple catchments to surface water models. In the unified transport model [80], the runoff and surface water models also are linked to an atmospheric transport model that estimates contaminant deposition on land and water. It should be noted that while the modeling of hydrological dep-processes in these models is quite detailed, contaminant/sediment partitioning, volatilization, and degradation often are modeled using the same partitioning coefficients and first-order rate constants employed by Mills et al. [69].

Surface Water Models

The objective of surface water modeling is to predict the movement, dilution, partitioning, and degradation of contaminants in surface water. Typical problems for which surface water models have been developed include estimation of (1) the position and size of plumes and/or mixing zones for point-source discharges, (2) the downstream movement rate, dispersion, and fate of contaminants following spills or other pulse discharge events, and (3) average concentrations as a function of distance, for continuous point-source or nonpoint-source discharges. As with runoff models, the basic driving forces in surface water models are the movement of water and sediment as determined by the law of conservation of mass and momentum. These basic physical principles are coupled with contaminant-specific estimates of sediment–water partitioning, volatilization, and transformation/degradation. As with runoff models, a variety of models with varying complexity, simulation capability, and information requirements have been developed.

The best known surface water model is the exposure analysis and modeling system (EXAMS) [7,17]. EXAMS represents a water body as a series of linked compartments, within which contaminants are sorbed and desorbed from particles, volatilized, and degraded. Each compartment is assumed to be homogeneous, and contaminant inputs are assumed to be constant. The number and types of compartments and the connections among them are defined by the model user. The outputs from EXAMS consist of estimates of steady-state contaminant concentrations in each compartment. EXAMS has been subjected to validation studies both in the laboratory [59] and in the field [33].

Although EXAMS employs simple steady-state hydrodynamics, it uses relatively complex environmental descriptions and process chemistry. Many removal processes are modeled as second-order, and multiple ionization states of a contaminant can be tracked simultaneously. To accommodate spatial variation in the rates of chemical processes, water bodies are vertically stratified and horizontally segmented according to four compartment types. Because the contaminant and site-specific information available for many assessment problems is insufficient to utilize the full capabilities of EXAMS, a number of scaled-down models employing the EXAMS concept have been developed. Mills et al. [69] describe simple analytical models for all types of surface water modeling problems, including rivers, lakes, and estuaries. It is assumed in these models that the systems are at steady-state (e.g., stream flows are not time-varying) and are either completely mixed or can be represented as a set of coupled, completely mixed segments. Various additional simplifying assumptions are used to develop models for different classes of rivers, lakes, and estuaries; readily evaluated classification criteria are provided for determining the appropriate model for a given system. DiToro et al. [26] describe a conceptually similar approach to modeling the fate of contaminants in lakes and rivers, including a detailed treatment of sediment–water partitioning, settling, and resuspension. Travis et al. [96] described a steady-state river model that computes statistical distributions of contaminant concentrations as functions of stochastically varying environmental parameters.

Many dynamic surface water models have been developed for use in situations where detailed simulation of contaminant distributions in space and time are desired. The basic principles and uses of dynamic surface water models are described in engineering textbooks [95]. In these models, the time-dependent equations of motion for water molecules, sediment particles, and contaminants are solved numerically. Examples include plume models for calculating contaminant or temperature distributions in the vicinities of point sources [55] and various water-quality simulation models [6,12]. The physical and chemical processes incorporated in these models are as those in steady-state models such as EXAMS; however, dynamic models can simulate the effects of time-varying contaminant inputs and hydrological parameters on contaminant concentrations in time and space.

Although a few three-dimensional models have been developed, most dynamic water quality models are one- or two-dimensional. Because the results obtained from dynamic models are highly site-dependent, they are designed for site-specific applications where detailed characterization of basin morphometry, background water quality, geochemistry, and hydrology is feasible.

Ground-water Transport

Rainfall that does not evaporate or run off infiltrates the soil. Hence, as a consequence of mass balance, many of the models developed for predicting contaminant runoff [69,75,80] also can predict infiltration of contaminated water into the soil. Except for multimedia models, such as the unified transport model [80], these models do not predict the rate of movement of contaminants through the unsaturated soil column to ground water. For this purpose, specialized models of hydrological processes in the soil column are needed. In addition to climatological characteristics (e.g., rainfall, temperature, and evapotranspiration), such models must account for soil characteristics (e.g., effective porosity, organic content, and permeability) as functions of soil depth. The best known model is SESOIL [11]. Given data on rates of contaminant deposition, site meteorology and soil characteristics in one to three layers, and contaminant-specific estimates of partitioning and degradation, SESOIL estimates steady-state rates of contaminant delivery to an aquifer underlying the unsaturated zone. Information on other unsaturated zone models can be obtained from a digitized data base compiled by the International Ground Water Modeling Center [50]. A different class of models is used to predict the movement of water and dissolved contaminants in aquifers. The rates of movement, dispersion, and diffusion of water and dissolved contaminants in saturated soil or rock are functions of hydraulic gradient, hydraulic conductivity, and effective porosity. Screening-level predictions of the rate and direction of movement of contaminants in ground water can be obtained from models based on analytical solutions to hydraulic equations in homogeneous media [20,28,31,74,102]. Many of these models account for the effects of degradation and retardation due to rock–solution partitioning. They are intended for use in predicting aquifer contaminant concentrations and travel times to order-of-magnitude accuracy.

Real subsurface environments are highly heterogeneous. Models of ground-water movement in heterogeneous media have been developed for use in evaluating the suitability of sites for underground disposal of hazardous wastes. In these models, the subsurface environment is divided into compartments with varying characteristics. Reviews of such models recently have been compiled [4,70,89]. Although spatially complex subsurface models allow realistic simulation of contaminant migration patterns, they require detailed site-specific hydrogeological surveys and may not be appropriate for assessing risks of bioengineered microorganisms applied to the vegetation or soil surface.

EVALUATION OF AVAILABLE METHODS FOR MODELING MICROBIAL TRANSPORT AND FATE

It is apparent from the above considerations that the capability for modeling the transport and fate of microbes in the environment varies considerably among pathways and organism types. Of the three pathways of primary interest in microbial fate assessment, suitable models appear available for two: aerial and waterborne transport. The fundamental force responsible for the transport of both microbes and hazardous chemical substances is the mass movement of air, water, and suspended particles. Many of the models developed for assessing environmental risks of radionuclides, pesticides, and toxic chemicals are, therefore, either directly applicable to or adaptable for use in assessing environmental risks of bioengineered microorganisms.

For atmospheric pathways, there is a very close correspondence between the processes governing the transport of microorganisms and those governing the transport of chemicals. The transport of airborne microbes, like that of particulate contaminants, depends primarily on dispersion, diffusion, and settling as functions of particle size. The same modeling approaches (e.g., Gaussian plume dispersion) have been employed in both. For aquatic pathways, the same physical processes control the transport of contaminants and microbes. However, the chemical processes responsible for sediment–water partitioning and volatilization of chemical contaminants are distinctly different from the analogous processes affecting microbial transport. Therefore, mechanistic models of contaminant partitioning and degradation in surface water and ground water are not applicable to microorganisms.

The environmental data required to model the transport of microbes are essentially the same data required to model the transport of chemical contaminants. However, the contaminant-specific data employed in these models must be replaced by microbe-specific data. As noted above, processes such as the partitioning of microbes between particles and solution, and the injection of microbes into the atmosphere from surface water, are not amenable to modeling by using the approaches developed for chemicals. Of even greater importance is the need for data on microbial survival. The terms in transport models corresponding to radioactive decay constants or contaminant degradation rates must be replaced by estimates of microbial death rates. It is evident that although many of the abiotic and biotic factors influencing microbial survival have been identified, few quantitative generalizations are possible.

There appear to be few, if any, existing models applicable to the third major transport pathway for bioengineered microorganisms: animal vectors. Models of pathogen dispersal via obligate animal hosts (e.g., mosquitoes) probably exist in the epidemiological literature, but these may not be applicable to modeling the passive dispersal of microorganisms by foraging or migrating animals.

CONCLUSIONS

Bacteria and viruses are readily transported in the environment by air, water, and animals. Existing models appear to be adequate for predicting the bulk transport of bioengineered microorganisms in air, surface water, and ground water. Such models are available for a wide range of spatiotemporal scales and assessment requirements. Models developed for plant pathogen assessment and contaminant fate assessment appear adequate for modeling the mass movement of microbes used in agriculture, sewage treatment, and pollution control. In all of these situations the release of a bioengineered microbe is analogous to the application of a pesticide, the dispersal of a naturally occurring pathogen, or the release of treated water from a sewage treatment plant.

Practical considerations suggest that, when selecting contaminant transport models for potential use in microbial risk assessments, it is desirable to emphasize models that are physics-intensive rather than chemistry-intensive. Model subroutines that estimate contaminant partitioning and degradation rates based on chemical kinetics are useless for quantifying microbial fate and may increase the difficulty of using the model. We recommend that the simpler of the existing models be used for predicting the transport of microorganisms by air and water. Examples of such models include the models described by Mills et al. [69] and Travis et al. [96]. We believe that risk assessments would not gain from the additional accuracy that is, in principle, achievable with high-resolution models. There seems little reason to require better than order of magnitude accuracy in dispersion estimates, given the much larger uncertainties regarding establishment, survival, and animal transport.

Transport of microbes by animals or man-made equipment is a unique phenomenon that has no counterpart in environmental chemistry, and existing models appear inadequate for modeling these pathways. Although the number of microorganisms carried by animal or technological vectors may be small, transport via these pathways is highly efficient. Animals can transport microorganisms rapidly over long distances. Moreover, there is a high probability that an animal carrying microbes away from a field or pond will travel to another field or pond suitable for colonization.

The key fate-related problems requiring research solutions are biological rather than physical or chemical. These include (1) the survival of microbes, especially in environments such as ground water, where direct observation is difficult, (2) the transport of microbes by animal vectors, and (3) the relationship between the number of viable microbes reaching a hospitable environment and the likelihood of their establishment and proliferation, and the spatial distribution of hospitable environments.

With respect to the above issues, the transport and establishment of microorganisms is more analogous to the migration and establishment of exotic plants and animals than to the transport and transformation of chemicals [90]. Predictive models of invasion and establishment, analogous to the contaminant fate models reviewed in this chapter, do not exist. However, biogeographic principles can be used to design experimental programs for evaluating the migration potential of introduced microorganisms, either on a case-by-case basis [91] or as part of a formal risk assessment protocol [94]. It appears that, although the physical aspects of microbial transport and fate in the environment are well-understood and can be adequately modeled, the biological aspects must be better-understood before models suitable for risk assessment can be developed.

Acknowledgments — The authors thank G. W. Suter II, C. C. Travis, and G. Stotz for comments on this paper. Research was sponsored by the U.S. Environmental Protection Agency under Interagency Agreement No. DW89930292-01-0 with the U.S. Department of Energy under Contract No. DE-AC05-840R21400 with Martin Marietta Energy Systems, Inc. Although the research described in this article has been funded wholly or in part by the United States Environmental Protection Agency (EPA) through Interagency Agreement No. DW89930292-01-0 to the U.S. Department of Energy, it has not been subjected to EPA review and therefore does not necessarily reflect the views of EPA and no official endorsement should be inferred. Publication No. 2588, Environmental Sciences Division, ORNL.

REFERENCES

1. Alexander, M. 1984. Fate and movements of microorganisms in the environment. Part 1. Survival and growth of bacteria. In J. W. Gillett, S. A. Levin, M. A. Harwell, D. A. Andow, and M. Alexander (Eds.), *Potential Impacts of Environmental Release of Biotechnology Products: Assessment, Regulation, and Research Needs*. Ecosystems Research Center, Cornell University, Ithaca, N.Y., pp. 47–62.

2. Andow, D. A. 1984. Fate and movement of microorganisms in the environment. Dispersal of microorganisms with novel genotypes. In J. W. Gillett, S. A. Levin, M. A. Harwell, D. A. Andow, and M. Alexander (Eds.), *Potential Impacts of Environmental Release of Biotechnology Products: Assessment, Regulation, and Research Needs*. Ecosystems Research Center, Cornell University, Ithaca, N.Y., pp. 88–103.

3. Babich, H. and G. Stozky. 1980. Environmental factors that influence the toxicity of heavy metals and gaseous pollutants to microorganisms. *Crit. Rev. Microbiol.* 8:99–145.

4. Bachmat, Y., B. Andrews, D. Holts, and S. Sebastian. 1978. Utilization of numerical ground water models for water resource management. EPA 600/8-78-012. U.S. Environmental Protection Agency, Environmental Research Laboratory, Ada, Okla.

5. Barnthouse, L. W., J. Boreman, S. W. Christensen, C. P. Goodyear, W. Van Winkle, and D. S. Vaughan. 1984. Population biology in the courtroom: The Hudson River controversy. *BioScience 34*:14–19.

6. Basta, D. J. and B. T. Bower. 1982. Analyzing natural systems: Analysis for regional residuals. Environmental Quality Management, Resources for the Future Inc. The Johns Hopkins University Press, Baltimore, Md.

7. Baughmann, G. L. and R. R. Lassiter. 1978. Prediction of environmental pollutant concentration. In J. Cairns, Jr., K. L. Dickson, and A. W. Maki (Eds.), *Estimating the Hazard of Chemical Substances to Aquatic Life*. ASTM STP 657. American Society for Testing and Materials, Philadelphia, pp. 35–54.

8. Bissonnette, G. K., J. J. Jezeski, G. A. McFeters, and D. G. Stuart. 1975. Influence of environmental stress on enumeration of indicator bacteria from natural waters. *Appl. Environ. Microbiol.* 29:186–194.

9. Bitton, G. and R. Mitchell. 1974. Effect of colloid on the survival of bacteriophages in seawater. *Water Res.* 8:227–229.

10. Bitton, G., S. R. Farrah, R. H. Ruskin, J. Butner, and Y. J. Chou. 1983. Survival of palogenic and indicator organisms in ground water. *Ground Water 21*:405–410.

11. Bonazountas, M. and J. Wagner. 1981. SESOIL: A seasonal soil compartment model. Draft report prepared by Arthur D. Little, Inc., Cambridge, Mass., for the U.S. Environmental Protection Agency, Office of Toxic Substances, Washington, D.C.

12. Boutwell, S. H. and B. R. Roberts. 1983. Assessment methodology for remedial actions in surface waters. Draft report prepared by Anderson-Nichols and Co., Palo Alto, Calif. for the U.S. Environmental Protection Agency Environmental Research Laboratory, Athens, Ga.

13. Bovallius, A., B. Bucht, R. Roffey, and P. Anas. 1978. Long-range air transmission of bacteria. *Appl. Environ. Microbiol.* 35:1231–1232.

14. Bovallius, A., R. Roffey, and E. Henningson. 1980. Long-range transmission of bacteria. *Ann. N.Y. Acad. Sci.* 353:186–200.

15. Brachman, P. S. 1980. Inhalation anthrax. *Ann. N.Y. Acad. Sci.* 353.83–93.

16. Braswell, J. R. and A. W. Hoadley. 1977. Recovery of *Escherichia coli* from chlorinated secondary sewage. *Appl. Microbiol.* 28:328–329.

17. Burns, L., R. Lassiter, and D. Cline. 1982. Documentation for the exposure assessment modeling system (EXAMS). EPA 600/3-82-023. U.S. Environmental Protection Agency Environmental Research Laboratory, Athens, Ga.

18. Carlucci, A. F. and D. Pramer. 1960. An evaluation of factors affecting the survival of *Escherichia coli* in sea water. Part II: Salinity, pH, and nutrients. *Appl. Microbiol.* 8:247–250.

19. Chen, M. and M. Alexander. 1973. Survival of soil bacteria during prolonged desiccation. *Soil Biol. Biochem.* 5:213–221.

20. Codell, R. B., K. T. Key, and G. Whelan. 1982. A collection of mathematical models for dispersion in surface water and ground water. NUREG-0868. U.S. Nuclear Regulatory Commission, Washington, D.C.

21. Costerton, J. W. 1984. Direct ultrastructural examination of adherent bacterial populations in natural and pathogenic ecosystems. In M. J. Klug and C. A. Reddy (Eds.), *Current Perspectives in Microbial Ecology.* American Society for Microbiology, Washington, D.C., pp. 115–123.

22. Crawford, N. H. 1982. Hydrologic transport modeling. In K. L. Dickson, A. W. Maki, and J. Cairns, Jr. (Eds.), *Modeling the Fate of Chemicals in the Aquatic Environment.* Ann Arbor Science Publishers, Ann Arbor, Mich., pp. 199–214.

23. Crosse, J. F. 1957. The dispersal of bacterial plant pathogens. In C. Horton Smith (Ed.), *Biological Aspects of the Transmission of Disease.* Oliver and Boyd, Edinburgh, Scotland, pp. 7–12.

24. Cuthbert, W. A., J. J. Panes, and E. C. Hill. 1950. Survival of *Bacterium coli* Type I and *Streptococcus faecalis* in soil. *J. Appl. Bacteriol.* 18:408.

25. Diesch, S. L. 1970. Disease transmission of water-borne organisms of animal origin. In T. L. Willrich and C. E. Smith (Eds.), *Agricultural Practices and Water Quality.* Iowa State University Press, Ames, Ia, pp. 265–285.

26. DiToro, D. M., D. J. O'Connor, R. V. Thomann, and J. P. St. John. 1982. Simplified model of the fate of partitioning chemicals in lakes and streams. In K. L. Dickson, A. W. Maki, and J. Cairns, Jr. (Eds.), *Modeling the Fate of Chemicals in the Aquatic Environment.* Ann Arbor Science Publishers, Ann Arbor, Mich., pp. 165–190.

27. Donigian, A. S., Jr. 1981. Water quality modeling in relation to watershed hydrology. In V. Singh (Ed.), *Modeling Components of Hydrologic Cycle.* Proceedings of the International Symposium on Rainfall Runoff Modeling. Mississippi State University. Water Resources Publications, Littleton, Colo.

28. Donigian, A. S., Jr., T. Y. R. Lo, and E. W. Shanahan. 1983. Rapid assessment of potential ground-water contamination under emergency response conditions. Draft report prepared by Anderson-Nicholls and Co., Palo Alto, Calif. for the U.S. Environmental Protection Agency Office of Health and Environmental Assessment, Washington, D.C.

29. Dorsey, E. L., R. F. Berenat, and E. L. Neff, Jr. 1970. Effect of sodium flores-cein and plating medium on recovery of irradiated *Escherichia coli* and *Serratia marcescens* from aerosols. *J. Appl. Microbiol. 20*:834–838.
30. Edmonds, R. L. 1976. Survival of coliform bacteria in sewage sludge applied to a forest clearcut and potential movement into groundwater. *Appl. Environ. Microbiol. 32*:537–546.
31. Enfield, G. G., R. F. Carsel, S. Z. Cohen, T. Phan, and D. M. Walters. 1982. Approximating pollutant transport to ground water. *Ground Water 20*:711–722.
32. Fletcher, M., and S. McEldowney. 1984. Microbial attachment to nonbiolog-ical surfaces. In M. J. Klug and C. A. Reddy (Eds.), *Current Perspectives in Microbial Ecology.* American Society for Microbiology, Washington, D.C., pp. 123–129.
33. Games, L. M. 1982. Field validation of exposure analysis modeling system (EXAMS) in a flowing stream. In K. L. Dickson, A. W. Maki, and J. Cairns, Jr. (Eds.), *Modeling the Fate of Chemicals in the Aquatic Environment.* Ann Arbor Science Publishers, Ann Arbor, Mich., pp. 325–346.
34. Geldreich, E. E. 1972. Water-borne pathogens. In R. M. Mitchell (Ed.), *Water Pollution Microbiology.* John Wiley and Sons, New York, pp. 207–241.
35. Gerba, C. P. 1984. Microorganisms as groundwater tracers. In G. Bitton and C. P. Gerba (Eds.), *Groundwater Pollution Microbiology.* John Wiley and Sons, New York, pp. 225–233.
36. Gerba, C. P. and G. Britton. 1984. Microbial pollutants: Their survival and transport pattern to ground water. In G. Britton and C. P. Gerba (Eds.), *Groundwater Pollution Microbiology.* John Wiley and Sons, New York, pp. 65–88.
37. Gerba, C. P., S. M. Goyal, I. Cech, and C. F. Bogdan. 1981. Quantitative assessment of the adsorptive behavior of viruses to soils. *Environ. Sci. Tech. 15*:940–944.
38. Germida, J. J. 1984. Persistence of nosema locustae spores in soils as determined by fluorescence microscopy. *Appl. Environ. Microbiol. 31*:605–608.
39. Gloster, J., R. M. Blackall, R. F. Sellers, and A. I. Donaldson. 1981. Forecast-ing the airborne spread of foot-and-mouth disease. *Vet. Record 108*:370–374.
40. Gregory, P. H. 1968. Interpreting plant disease dispersal gradients. *Ann. Rev. Phytopathol. 6*:189–212.
41. Gregory, P. H. 1973. *The Microbiology of the Atmosphere.* 2nd ed. John Wiley and Sons, New York.
42. Habte, M. and M. Alexander. 1977. Further evidence for the regulation of bac-terial populations in soil by protozoa. *Arch. Microbiol. 113*:181–183.
43. Hagedorn, C. 1984. Microbial aspects of groundwater pollution due to septic tanks. In G. Britton and C. P. Gerba (Eds.), *Groundwater Pollution Microbi-ology.* John Wiley and Sons, New York, pp. 181–196.
44. Harris, K. F. and K. Maramorosch. 1980. *Vectors of Plant Pathogens.* Aca-demic Press, New York.
45. Harrington, J. B. 1979. Principles of deposition of microbial particles. In R. L. Edmonds (Ed.), *Aerobiology: the Ecological Systems Approach.* Dowden, Hutchinson and Ross, Stroudsburg, Pa., pp. 111–137.
46. Heffter, J. L. and A. D. Taylor. 1975. A regional-continental scale transport, diffusion, and deposition model. Part I: Trajectory model. NOAA Technical Memorandum ERL-ARL-50. Air Resources Laboratories, Silver Spring, Md.
47. Hoffman, F. O., D. L. Schaeffer, C. W. Miller, and C. T. Garten, Jr., Eds. 1978. Proceedings of a workshop on the evaluation of models used for the envi-

ronmental assessment of radionuclide releases. CONF-770901. Oak Ridge National Laboratory, Oak Ridge, Tenn.

48. Hug, A., P. A. West, E. B. Small, M. I. Hug, and R. R. Colwell. 1984. Influence of water temperature, salinity, and pH on survival and growth of toxigenic *Vibrio cholerae* Serovar 01 associated with live copepods in laboratory microcosms. *Appl. Environ. Microbiol.* 48:420–424.

49. Hydrocomp International, Inc. 1979. User's manual for the hydrological simulation program — FORTRAN (HSPF). U.S. Environmental Protection Agency Environmental Research Laboratory, Athens, Ga.

50. International Ground Water Modeling Center 1982. Mass transport models which are documented and currently available. GWM 82-02. Holcomb Research Institute, Butler University, Indianapolis, Ind.

51. Kibbey, H. J., C. Hagedorn, and E. L. McCoy. 1978. Use of fecal *streptococci* as indicators of pollution in soil. *Appl. Environ. Microbiol.* 35:711–717.

52. Kjelleberg, S. 1984. Effects of interfaces on survival mechanisms of copiotrophic bacteria in low-nutrient habitats. In M. J. Klug and C. A. Reddy (Eds.), *Current Perspectives in Microbial Ecology*. American Society for Microbiology, Washington, D.C., pp. 151–159.

53. Klein, D. A. and L. E. Casida, Jr. 1967. *Escherichia coli* die-out from normal soil as related to nutrient availability and the indigenous microflora. *Can. J. Microbiol.* 13:1461–1470.

54. Ko, W. H. and F. K. Chow. 1977. Characteristics of bacteriostasis in natural soils. *J. Gen. Microbiol.* 102:295–298.

55. Koh, R. C. Y. and L. N. Fan. 1970. Mathematical models for the prediction of temperature distributions resulting from the discharge of heated water into large bodies of water. Water Pollution Control Series 16/30 DWD 10/70. U.S. Environmental Protection Agency, Washington, D.C.

56. Lance, J. C. and C. P. Gerba. 1984. Virus movement in soil during saturated and unsaturated flow. *Appl. Environ. Microbiol.* 47:335-337.

57. Lange, R. 1975. ADPIC, a three-dimensional transport-diffusion model for the dispersal of atmospheric pollutants and its validation against regional tracer studies. UCRL-76170. Lawrence Livermore Laboratory, Livermore, Calif.

58. Langmuir, A. D. 1980. Changing concepts of airborne infection of acute contagious diseases: A reconsideration of classic epidemiologic theories. *Ann. N.Y. Acad. Sci.* 353:35–44.

59. Lassiter, R. R. 1982. Testing models of the fate of chemicals in aquatic environments. In K. L. Dickson, A. W. Maki, and J. Cairns, Jr. (Eds.), *Modeling the Fate of Chemicals in the Aquatic Environment*. Ann Arbor Science Publishers, Ann Arbor, Mich., pp. 287–301.

60. LeChevallier, M. W., S. C. Cameron, and G. A. McFeters. 1983. New medium for improved recovery of coliform bacteria from drinking water. *Appl. Environ. Microbiol.* 45:484–492.

61. Liang, L. N., J. L. Sinclair, L. M. Mallory, and M. Alexander. 1982. Fate in model ecosystems of microbial species of potential use in genetic engineering. *Appl. Environ. Microbiol.* 44:708–714.

62. Lighthart, B. and A. S. Frisch. 1976. Estimation of viable airborne microbes downwind from a point source. *Appl. Environ. Microbiol.* 31:700–704.

63. Lighthart, B., J. C. Spendlove, and T. G. Akers. 1979. Sources and characteristics of airborne materials: Bacteria and viruses. In R. L. Edmonds (Ed.), *Aerobiology: The Ecological Systems Approach*. Dowden, Hutchinson, and Ross, Stroudsburg, Pa., pp. 11–12.

64. Linderman, J. and C. D. Upper. 1985. Aerial dispersal of epiphytic bacteria over bean plants. *Appl. Environ. Microbiol.* 50:1229–1232.

65. Lowe, W. E. and T. R. G. Gray. 1973. Ecological studies on coccoid bacteria in a pine forest soil. Part II: Growth of bacteria introduced into soil. *Soil Biol. Biochem.* 5:449–462.

66. Maguire, B., Jr. 1963. The passive dispersal of small aquatic organisms and their colonization of isolated bodies of water. *Ecol. Monogr.* 33:161–185.

67. Mallman, W. L. and W. Litsky. 1951. Survival of selected enteric organisms in various types of soil. *Am. J. Pub. Health* 41:38–44.

68. Maramorosch, K. and K. F. Harris. 1981. *Plant Diseases and Vectors: Ecology and Epidemiology.* Academic Press, New York.

69. Mills, W. B., J. D. Dean, D. B. Porcella, S. A. Gherini, R. J. M. Hudson, W. E. Frick, G. L. Rupp, and G. L. Bowie. 1982. Water quality assessment: A screening procedure for toxic and conventional pollutants. EPA-600/6-82-004 (2 vols.). U.S. Environmental Protection Agency Environmental Research Laboratory, Athens, Ga.

70. Moiser, J. E., J. R. Fowler, C. J. Barton, W. W. Tolbert, S. C. Myers, J. E. Vancil, H. A. Price, M. J. R. Vasdo, E. E. Rutz, T. X. Wendeln, and L. D. Rickertson. 1980. Low-level waste management: A compilation of models and monitoring techniques. ORNL/SMB-79/13617/2. Science Applications, Inc., Oak Ridge, Tenn.

71. Moore, R. E., et al. 1979. AIRDOS-EPA: A computerized methodology for estimating environmental concentrations and dose to man from airborne releases of radionuclides. EPA-520/1-79-009, U.S. Environmental Protection Agency Office of Radiation Programs, Washington, D.C.

72. Murphy, B. D., S. Y. Ohr, and C. L. Begovich. 1984. RETADD-II: A long-range atmospheric trajectory model with consistent treatment of deposition loss and species growth and decay. ORNL/CSD-99. Oak Ridge National Laboratory, Oak Ridge, Tenn.

73. Nabbut, N. H. and F. Kurayiyya. 1972. Survival of *Salmonella* typhi in seawater. *J. Hyg.* 70:223–228.

74. Nelson, R. W. and J. A. Schur. 1980. Paths ground-water hydrologic model. PNL-3162. Battelle, Pacific Northwest Laboratories, Richland, Wash.

75. Onishi, Y., S. M. Brown, A. R. Olsen, M. A. Parkhurst, S. E. Wise, and W. H. Walters. 1982. Methodology for overland and instream migration and risk assessment of pesticides. EPA-600/3-82-024. U.S. Environmental Protection Agency Environmental Research Laboratory, Athens, Ga.

76. Osa-Afiana, L. O. and M. Alexander. 1979. Effect of moisture on survival of *Rhizobium* in soil. *Soil Sci. Soc. Am. J.* 43:925–930.

77. Osa-Afiana, L. O. and M. Alexander. 1982. Differences among cowpea *Rhizobia* in tolerance to high temperature and dessication in soil. *Appl. Environ. Microbiol.* 43:435–439.

78. Paerl, H. W. and K. K. Gallucci. 1985. Role of chemotaxis in establishing a specific nitrogen-fixing cyanobacter-bacterial association. *Science* 227:647–649.

79. Parhad, N. M. and N. U. Rao. 1974. Effect of pH on survival of *Escherichia coli. J. Water Pollut. Cont. Fed.* 46:980–986.

80. Patterson, M. R., T. J. Sworski, A. L. Sjoreen, M. G. Browman, C. C. Coutant, D. M. Hetrick, B. D. Murphy, and R. J. Raridon. 1983. A user's manual for UTM-TOX: The unified transport model. ORNL/TM-8182. Oak Ridge National Laboratory, Oak Ridge, Tenn.

81. Peterson, E. W. and B. Lighthart. 1977. Estimation of downwind viable air-

borne microbes from a wet cooling tower, including settling. *Microbial. Ecol.* 4:67–79.

82. Porges, R. and K. M. Mackenthun. 1963. Waste stabilization ponds: Use, function, and biota. *Biotech. Bioeng.* 5:255–273.

83. Pringle, J. H. and M. Fletcher. 1983. Influence of substratum wettability on attachment of freshwater bacteria to solid surfaces. *Appl. Environ. Microbiol.* 45:811–817.

84. Raridon, R. J., B. D. Murphy, W. M. Culkowski, and M. R. Patterson. (in press). The atmospheric transport model as applied to toxic substances (ATM-TOX). ORNL/CSD-94. Oak Ridge National Laboratory, Oak Ridge, Tenn.

85. Romero, J. C. 1970. The movement of bacteria and viruses through porous media. *Ground Water* 8:37–48.

86. Rheinheimer, G. 1980. *Aquatic Microbiology.* John Wiley and Sons, New York.

87. Schaad, N. W. and W. C. White. 1974. Survival of *Xanthomonas campestris* in soil. *Ann. Rev. Phytopath.* 64:1518–1520.

88. Schroth, M. N., S. V. Thomson, D. C. Hildebrand, and W. J. Moller. 1974. Epidemiology and control of fire blight. *Ann. Rev. Phytopathol.* 12:389–412.

89. Science Applications, Inc. 1981. Tabulation of Waste Isolation Computer Models. ONWI-78. Office of Nuclear Waste Isolation, Battelle Memorial Institute, Columbus, Ohio.

90. Sharples, F. E. 1983. Spread of organisms with novel genotypes: thoughts from an ecological perspective. *Recombinant DNA Technol. Bull.* 6:43–56.

91. Simberloff, D. 1985. Predicting ecological effects of novel entities: evidence from higher organisms. In H. O. Halvorson, D. Pramer, and M. Rogul (Eds.), *Engineered Organisms in the Environment: Scientific Issues.* American Society for Microbiology, Washington, D.C., pp. 152–161.

92. Sinclair, J. M. and M. Alexander. 1984. Role of resistance to starvation in bacterial survival in sewage and lake water. *Appl. Environ. Microbiol.* 48:410–415.

93. Slade, D. H. (Ed.). 1968. Meteorology and atomic energy – 1968. TID-24190, Environmental Sciences Services Administration. U.S. Atomic Energy Commission, Washington, D.C.

94. Suter, G. W. II. 1985. Application of environmental risk analysis to engineered organisms. In H. O. Halvorson, D. Pramer, and M. Rogul (Eds.), *Engineered Organisms in the Environment: Scientific Issues.* American Society for Microbiology, Washington, D.C., pp. 211–219.

95. Thomann, R. V. 1972. *Systems Analysis and Water Quality Management.* McGraw-Hill, New York.

96. Travis, C. C., C. F. Baes III, L. W. Barnthouse, E. L. Etnier, C. A. Holton, B. D. Murphy, G. P. Thompson, G. W. Suter II, and A. P. Watson. 1983. Exposure assessment methodology and reference environments for synfuel risk analysis. ORNL/TM-8672. Oak Ridge National Laboratory, Oak Ridge, Tenn.

97. U.S. Environmental Protection Agency. 1977. User's manual for single source (CRSTER) model. EPA-450/2-77-013. U.S. Environmental Protection Agency Office of Air Quality Planning and Standards, Research Triangle Park, N.C.

98. Van Donsel, D. J., E. E. Geldreich, and N. A. Clarke. 1967. Seasonal variations of indicator bacteria in soil and their contribution to storm-water pollution. *Appl. Environ. Microbiol.* 15:1362–1370.

99. Williams, J. R. 1975. Sediment-yield prediction with universal equation using runoff energy factor. In *Present and Prospective Technology for Predicting Sediment Yields and Sources.* ARS-s-40. U.S. Department of Agriculture, Washington, D.C.

100. Wischmeier, W. H. and D. D. Smith. 1965. Predicting rainfall-erosion losses from cropland east of the Rocky Mountains. Agriculture Handbook ARS-282. U.S. Department of Agriculture, Washington, D.C.
101. Wolman, A. and A. E. Gorman. 1931. *The Significance of Waterborne Typhoid Fever Outbreaks, 1920-1930*. Williams and Wilkins, Baltimore, Md.
102. Yeh, G. T. 1981. Analytical transient one-, two-, and three-dimensional (AT123D) simulation of waste transport in the aquifer system. ORNL-5602. Oak Ridge National Laboratory, Oak Ridge, Tenn.
103. Young, C. C. and H. Greenfield. 1923. Observations on the viability of the *Bacterium coli* group under natural and artificial conditions. *Am. J. Pub. Health 13*:270–273.
104. Zobell, C. E. 1942. Microorganisms in marine air. In S. Moulton (Ed.), *Aerobiology*. Publication No. 17 American Association of Advanced Science, Washington, D.C., pp. 55–68.

Ecosystem Structural
and Functional Analysis

Richard G. Wiegert

A starting point for a risk analysis of the release into the environment of genetically engineered organisms is to analyze the probable effects on the structural and functional attributes of the target ecosystem(s). Although this analysis could lead logically to a full mechanistic model incorporating known information on structure and function, much can be said on the basis of a simpler first-pass analysis.

Structure and function are used commonly in the ecological literature, but their meanings seldom are given explicitly. Indeed, ecology itself is sometimes described as the study of the structure and function of nature [5]. In this ecological context, function usually is thought of as what the system does and structure is what allows the system to do it. Thus, structural parameters of the ecosystem identify the "things" in the system, for example, species, numerical density, and biomass. Functional parameters comprise energy flows, nutrient cycling, and regulatory processes. The difficulties inherent in these ecological definitions, from the standpoint of systems analysis, become apparent if we contrast them with the systems theory concepts of structure and function.

In systems theory, what the system does, that is, what it produces in the way of observable "output," is regarded as behavior, and the means whereby the behavior is produced are provided by the interaction of system structure with system-functional attributes [3]. We can observe the behaviors of ecosystems, but the intergradation of system structure and function is usually so tight that these behaviors are not distinguished by most measurements. However, they can be represented separately in mathematical models of the system. In Figure 7.1, the model is represented by components, each comprising a box and its contents. The flows between them are indicated by a directional arrow and the nature of the interaction — that is, F(X, Y, T, P), a function of state variables X; Y; T, time; and P, parameters. In section (a) of the figure, two different arrangements of these four parts illustrate the distinction between the systems theoretical and the ecological usages of structure and function. Systems structure corresponds to the boxes and the arrows connecting them. Systems function, on the other hand, is defined as the time-varying contents of the compartments. For example, function comprises the values of the state variables through time and the form of the interactions, that is, the magnitude of the fluxes and the form of the control functions. These values in turn depend on the component state variables X and Y, as well as on P and T, as shown in section (b). The ecological definitions are given in section (c), where the abstract boxes (niches) and their occupants are considered structural and both the arrows and the form of the interactions are regarded as functional attributes of the system.

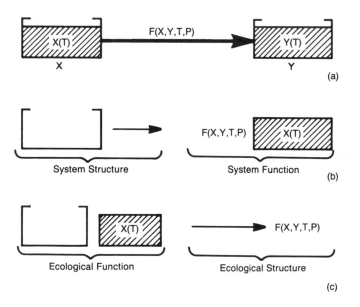

Figure 7.1. Identification of structure and function in a system diagram. (From Hill and Wiegert [3].)

The systems view of structure and function offers several operational advantages in the analysis of system behavior and thus in the assessment of risk. For one thing, the system structure is a much more enduring property than system function. That is, the replacement of a species or change in its physiological characteristics does not necessarily alter its structural position or connections with other components of the ecosystem. Second, in many ecosystems it is much easier to identify gross structural properties of the system than to estimate functional attributes; thus, the assessment of structural change is easier. Although ecosystem structure is, by itself, an incomplete specification of a system, useful models can often be constructed with a minimum of time and expense if an accurate picture of ecosystem structure is fleshed out with a sharply constrained set of functional parameters, or even with qualitative information about component interactions.

Viewed in this way, any assessment of the probable effects of introducing bioengineered organisms must first address the question of whether there is a possibility of structural changes (new predator–prey or parasite–host relationships), functional changes (organisms responding differently to their environment), or both. Answers to this question depend on decisions about how likely the effects are to be important (and thus how much time and money is justified in their evaluation), and just where in the system they are expected to manifest themselves. In particular, since there are many types of structural arrows denoting input–output relationships (e.g., those depicting informational flow), structural analysis of a system provides a starting point for distinguishing between the fate (destination) of matter and energy inputs and their rate of transport. This structural analysis can be expanded to include qualitative aspects of function and employed as a useful tool to assess some ecological consequences of releases of biologically engineered organisms into the ecosystem.

STEPS IN ECOSYSTEM ANALYSIS

The methods of ecosystem analysis include (1) specification of compartments (state variables), (2) specification of the network, or matter and energy transfers (i.e., arrows), (3) specification of transfers of information causing regulation or control of the flows of matter and energy, and (4) the qualitative and quantitative evaluation of functional attributes of the ecosystem. In a very general way, the potential sensitivity of the structure or function as well as the difficulty of evaluation increases from methods 1 through 4. Most of the following discussion is confined to methods 1 through 3. Evaluation of functional attributes of specific occupants of structural compartments of ecosystems is developed further in chapter 5 of this volume.

Specification of Compartmental Structure

The first requirement is to have sufficient knowledge of the system potentially at risk so that a set of significant components can be identified. In this context, "significant" is defined in part by the value system held by the investigators in connection with the type of organisms to be released. This section only sketches methods in principle, using highly aggregated compartments. Any combination of less aggregated components could be substituted by appropriate decomposition of a compartment and its flows. Similarly, compartments, connections, and processes will be examined solely from the standpoint of potential effects of the release of exotic microorganisms.

In constructing the component or "box" structure of the system, some of the energy notation of Odum [6] is useful.

A "bullet" shape represents an autotrophic compartment, able to fix carbon through the use of solar energy (or an inorganic chemical source of energy).

A "tank" represents an abiotic storage component.

A "hexagon" represents a heterotrophic consumer component.

The relative size of the figures can be used in the structural diagram to provide an indication of relative standing stock or importance.

A structural diagram of a representative terrestrial ecosystem is shown in Figure 7.2 with sufficient detail of flow and information transfer to permit discussion of methods for analysis.

We can evaluate importance of the components on the basis of several different criteria. Standing stock serves as a prominent and rather easily determined attribute for most system components. In Figure 7.2 the relative size of the woody plant (shoots plus roots) and the particulate organic carbon components are represented as important (based on biomass). This criterion, however, provides the least satisfactory measure of importance for a structural analysis from the standpoint of biorisk, because it gives no indication of susceptibility to perturbation and because compartment size is often a less satisfactory indicator of importance than the flow of matter and energy.

Thus, the second criterion to be applied to the structural component diagram is the degree to which the component is susceptible to perturbation, that is, its "vulnerability." High susceptibility coupled with a large biomass is much more significant than either criterion alone. However, implementing this second criterion requires substantially more detailed knowledge of the system than a simple biomass-based estimate, because vulnerability is really a systems-level property whose evaluation requires knowledge of function as well as structure. For example, in Figure 7.2 the highly ag-

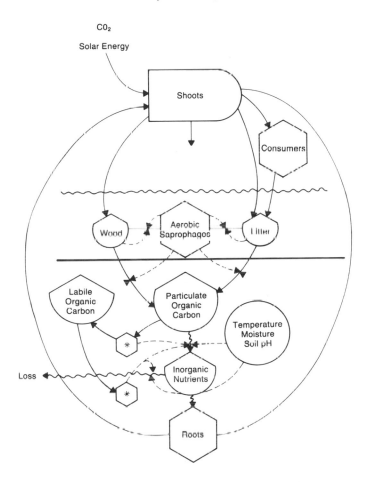

Figure 7.2. Structural diagram of a representative aggregated terrestrial ecosystem. A few of the important pathways of carbon/energy flow (——) and material cycling (⌣) are diagrammed, together with the transfers of information (———) responsible for regulation and control. CO_2 respiration/heat sink from each component is implied. The asterisks indicate anaerobic saprophages (microbes).

gregated nature of the autotrophic component (shoots vs. roots) provides little basis for an evaluation of how susceptible the woody plants might be to the introduction of a microorganism potentially able to infect trees, because most such parasites (e.g., oak wilt, Dutch elm disease, chestnut blight) are specific to one or a limited number of closely related species of tree. Thus, the autotrophic component diagram (Fig. 7.2) would have to be increased in detail to at least the genus level to consider a susceptibility criterion. This is to say nothing of the information that would have to be obtained about the biological capabilities of the bioengineered organism. In the example used, woody plant flora are rather easily assessed; in the case of other aggregated components, however, particularly those dominated by microorganisms, the difficulties could be insurmountable, given the present state of knowledge concerning the composition of microbial communities in the field.

Specification of the Network of Matter/Energy Flow Pathways

The next step in an ecosystem structural analysis is to include arrows showing the pathway and direction of transfers of matter and energy among the components of the system (see Fig. 7.2). These arrows provide some additional criteria for evaluating the importance of the components.

The utility of the structural diagram is greatly enhanced if it illustrates that the component in question is unique in the sense that no other component in the system does or could occupy the same trophic position — thus ensuring that if the specified pathway were blocked, the blockage would be permanent. Clearly this would be a potentially more serious consequence of perturbation and thus elevate the importance of the component in the assessment of risk of flow interruption. Another problem is the risk of a potentially damaging or dangerous organism establishing a new pathway in the system.

Finally, the structural diagram allows the connectedness of the entire system to be evaluated. Thus, for the first time in the step-by-step development of the structural diagram, we have a measure of the susceptibility of the system as a whole, rather than only a set of measures for each component. The connectedness of the system can be described as the number of pathways in the system and expressed as a percentage of the computed maximum number possible. For a system of n components, the maximum is $n^2 - n$ or, if the two possible paths between each component and the surrounding environment are included, $n^2 + n$. This figure, together with the number of components, gives some idea of the complexity of the system and thus permits some observations concerning its relative stability. This is, however, an extremely simplified view of connectedness. For example, we might wish to separate state-variable path connections according to whether they convey both matter and energy (and thus some information) or only information (feedback control). The latter pathways in particular may operate only part of the time and under conditions imposed by the system components. When expressing connectedness, we might also take into account the relative strength of each connection (i.e., some measure of its importance), which would overlap with measures of system function.

For decades there has been a controversy in ecology concerning the relationship between diversity, whether measured as simple species number or with some estimate of connectedness as complexity, and stability. Whether diversity confers stability or, as suggested by Smith [8], the stability of an ecosystem is necessary for the evolution of diversity, the fact remains that diversity and stability are correlated in the majority of natural systems observed. Unfortunately, the same relationship does not hold for model systems. Increasing connectance, for example, often does not confer stability on model systems. When increasing the complexity of model ecosystems by adding connections, the stability of the models is at best not affected, and may actually decrease [7]. Gardner and Ashby [2] showed that increasing connectedness slowly decreased stability up to a critical percentage, following which stability decreased rapidly. A partial resolution of this apparent paradox between model systems and the real world is the observation that stable and complex real-world systems may represent those few configurations of complexity and stability observable in model systems; all other configurations possible, being inherently unstable, are not seen in nature, having become extinct [4].

A nice resolution of this seeming paradox is found in the measure of "ascendancy" proposed by Ulanowicz [9]. Briefly, the ascendancy of the system is the product of the total system network (in whatever units the latter is measured), and trophic organization is measured as the information content, in a manner analogous to the H species diversity function. As a trophic network develops, that is, reduces redundant pathways, its information content and ascendancy increase, but its vulnerability to perturbation increases. The amount of possible information increases with the number of compartments. Thus, stable systems with many compartments may have proceeded to a high level of development (high ascendancy) and have a redundancy that is small as a percentage of developmental capacity, although large in absolute terms. The redundant pathways in such systems are not provided randomly; rather, they exist as the result of long evolutionary development, under strong selective pressure. In an analogous manner, although randomly adding pathways does not stabilize a model and may often destabilize one, selectively added pathways can stabilize.

The lesson here is that using component number and connectance to provide a measure of system stability in the face of a biotic perturbation must be done with extreme caution. To the extent that the structural model is a reasonable facsimile of the real system in number of components and detail of trophic connections, complexity may be an indication of stability.

Information Transfer Leading to Regulation/Control

The structural system diagram is completed by adding the network of pathways of information transfer, which are the basis for the control and regulation of matter and energy in the system. Without such controls, no system can exist, for each component would either grow without limit or decline to zero.

In the model system given in Figure 7.2, the network of pathways is as follows: the autotrophic component fixes carbon; translocates to the roots; is fed upon by the consumers of leaves and wood; and in autumn (assuming for the moment a deciduous system) drops leaves and, upon the death of limbs or trunks, wood to the litter zone. Figure 7.2 shows the matter–energy transfers and a few of the significant informational transfers that have to do with microbial transformers in the litter and soil. Transformation of litter and wood to the forms of particulate organic carbon found in the soil is governed in large part by aerobic saprophages, bacteria, and especially fungi, which use part of the energy to effect the transformation. These also produce more labile organic organisms that in turn provide energy-rich substrates for the anaerobic forms found in the soil. Some of the latter decompose the particulate organic carbon directly, releasing some additional organic elements and also facilitating the leaching of inorganic elements (nutrients) from the large pool of organic matter. Other anaerobic forms use labile organic energy substrates and transform the inorganic nutrients into forms assimilable by the plant roots. These microbes may also, by either actions, promote or control the loss of inorganic nutrients from the system or even result in gains, such as a nitrogen fixation.

Clearly, the most vulnerable points in any such system to the perturbation caused by the introduction of a new organism would be controls affecting the flows from components judged on the basis of the earlier measures to be important to the system. Although the structure of the control and regulation attribute of any given system provides the best and most sensitive measure of its probable response in acute or chronic perturbation, this attribute unfortunately is difficult and expensive to ascertain. There are few ecosystems managed by humans, and even fewer natural systems, for which we have more than a rudimentary idea of the structure of the control network. Although the example given in Figure 7.2 is highly simplified when compared to any real ecosystem, it does present some essential points. For example, in almost every terrestrial ecosystem of which we have knowledge, and in many aquatic systems as well, the decomposer community is so important that its complete failure would result in drastic changes in the system in a matter of years. Indeed, it is estimated that the annual worldwide turnover of carbon by decomposers is on the order of 4 % of the total atmospheric carbon content.

Most ecosystems are *detritus* systems which means that most (often more than 90 %) of the net primary production is not consumed in the living state, but instead dies and is utilized as detritus. Because of the dominance of microorganisms in many stages of this utilization, we see another reason why this group could be so important in biorisk analysis. But microorganisms cannot always act alone, or at least the decomposition rates would be far lower without the intervention of invertebrates and sometimes vertebrates. The larger detritus feeders are particularly necessary in mesic and arid environments, where detritus tends to dry out more rapidly [1].

By placing a sign on information-flow arrows indicating the direction of action of a control factor, the analysis of probable effect can be facilitated further. For example, the arrow indicating a transfer of energy from litter to aerobic saprophages (Figure 7.2) suggests that increased litter has a positive effect on the movement of energy. If the influence of aerobic saprophages on the movement of energy from litter to particulate organic carbon is positive, then increasing litter and thus increasing aerobic saprophages would in turn accelerate the transformation of litter to humus— a positive feedback. In most cases, however, the positive arrow on the matter–energy pathway does not show the complete or final story, particularly when the transfer is from an abiotic or biotic component to a biotic one. Biotic components that are capable of autocatalytic growth under suitable conditions typically are regulated by functions that contain thresholds, thus introducing discontinuities into the equations representing the flows of matter and energy. The net result is that an increase in litter will have a positive effect on flow of material from litter to aerobic saprophages only if the amount of litter is not so great that it saturates the ability of the saprophages to utilize it. Similarly, aerobic saprophages may not always have a positive effect on the transformation of litter to particulate organic carbon in the soil, particularly when the supply of litter is low and much of it is utilized for energy by the saprophages. Furthermore, the precise effect of an increase or decrease in any particular component also depends on the form of the regulatory function (see below). Thus, the modification or loss of a particular control pathway will produce effects on a compartment's standing stocks and on the magnitude of flows, which will have to be evaluated on the basis of the extent of the control, and in particular on its functional form.

The form of the feedback functions reflects the verbal description of how the particular flow is controlled. The ecological literature is replete with specific mathematical formulations that represent the way in which organisms respond to changes in the availability of their resources or other changes in their environment. Unfortunately, there has been little attempt, even in the modeling literature, to systematize these forms and to make them realistically reflect the way organisms actually behave. In large part, this neglect appears to have arisen from the dominance of the theoretical literature by those more interested in the mathematical manipulation of models than in simulating the behavior of real systems. Thus, the following summary defines a general approach to the control of matter and energy flow that permits the use of any realistic control function.

The specific example is a description of how to define two realistic control functions for a flow into a biotic component, that is, ingestion, since this type of flow exhibits the greatest variety in the way in which it is controlled in different groups of organisms. For a fuller description of this approach and citations of earlier publications, see Wiegert, Wetzel, and Christian [11].

Ingestion of matter and energy can be represented as a transfer from component x_1 to component x_2 or F_{12}:

$$F_{12} = x_2 \cdot t_{12} \cdot f(x_1) \cdot f(x_2)$$

where t_{12} = maximum specific rate of ingestion of matter/energy

$f(x_1)$ = the reduction of t_{12} due to scarcity of a material resource (measured in the units used for bookkeeping in the model)

$f(x_2)$ = the reduction of t_{12} due to scarcity of space

The requirement of this equation, since t_{12} is defined as the maximum possible rate under the conditions defined, is that both $f(x_1)$ and $f(x_2)$ take values between 0 and 1. When conditions are optimal with respect to both food and space, both control functions take the value 1, and the equation reduces to $F_{12} = x_2 \cdot t_{12}$. It is generally desirable to define $f(x_2)$ such that when the density of x_2 reaches some specified value, defined as the carrying capacity with respect to space alone, food being optimally available, then $f(x_2) \cdot t_{12}$ is equal to the sum of all minimal rates of loss, such as respiration, excretion, and physiological mortality. Then ingestion equals losses and $dx_2/dt = 0$.

Using the approach suggested by the previously shown equation, the control functions may be defined in any way that is consistent with how the components behave with respect to changes in the limiting resources. Even the maximum rate need not be a constant, but can be replaced with any variable that might improve the realism of the model. The simplest relationship between the limiting factor and realized specific rate of ingestion is a linear one, whereby a unit change in the availability of the limiting factor (x_1 or x_2 in the above example) has the same effect on the realized rate of ingestion, whether the unit change took place when the factor was scarce or abundant. In order that the control functions never exceed 1, an upper threshold level must be inserted in the function. In the case of food, further increases have no effect above a satiation level. This realistic effect is lacking in most functions used in ecological models. Often a lower threshold level is called for as well. In the case of the space function, this is a density below which organisms no longer compete for space.

The form of the control functions, linear or nonlinear, together with the normal value of the variable exerting the limiting or control effect, will determine the effect of modifying or eliminating the function as a consequence of the introduction of an exotic organism. With many microorganisms, in particular those commonly found adhering to and feeding from or penetrating surfaces, the control functions that best express the real situation key on thresholds that are not absolute densities or abundances, but which instead are ratios of abundance of the donor-limiting substrate and the recipient organism, as both a material resource and a living space [10].

Specifying the form of the control functions brings us to the border between structural and functional attributes of a system. To the extent that all species members of a component share the same general form of a control function, that is, they respond similarly to changes in the availability of the limiting factor, the form of the control function is a structural attribute. Whether this requirement of similar response is met is dependent on the aggregation of the structural components. Generally, the structural analysis will have to be subdivided finely enough so that functional forms for the feedback controls can be specified along with the compartment. When it comes to delineating parameters of the model, however, we definitely leave the structural realm and begin a functional description.

Qualitative and Quantitative Evaluation of Functional Attributes

The functional characteristics of the occupants of the structurally defined components are used in conjunction with the structural attributes in any risk assessment for a real ecosystem. If, for example, some aspects of the system function are known, specifically the fluxes of matter and energy, a measure of functional importance somewhat analogous to the structural biomass measure is possible.

Thus, the preceding discussion of structural analysis — enumeration of components, delineation of trophic transfers of matter and energy, specification of information transfer and of the form of the control and regulatory functions — cannot provide more than a very general assessment of the probable effects of release. Whether a released organism will survive and grow in a given ecosystem and have an impact on the system depends on the characteristics of the released organism and those of the organisms in the target system. All that can be inferred from the structural analysis alone, given that the organism survives and multiplies, are the probable components, flows, or controls with which it might interfere and the qualitative results that might be expected from the standpoint of the whole system.

EVALUATION OF METHODS

Compartment Structure and Flow Networks

Because of the active pursuit of descriptive ecology since the early decades of this century, there is a rather large body of knowledge available on the component structure and pathways of the flow of matter and energy in a wide variety of ecosystems. Such descriptions are widespread enough that further purely descriptive work can be done very selectively with regard to areas of the world, or parts of ecosystems, based on esthetic or economic value, and on potential importance in terms of high vulnerability of impact by bioengineered microorganisms.

The unfortunate aspect of this wealth of information about man-made as well as natural ecosystems is that it is concentrated in aspects of the system that, at least in the initial stages of biotechnology, are at little risk from introduced microorganisms or unimportant from the standpoint of an effect being spread throughout the system. As mentioned in the earlier example (Fig. 7.2), any one released organism would probably not irretrievably damage all of the important above-ground autotrophs or their heterotrophic grazers, because of the high diversity found in such systems. The same cannot be said for man-managed systems, at least in well-developed countries, because these countries typically favor low-diversity systems. Nevertheless, the most important part of an ecosystem, in terms of its significance to all aspects of system structure and function, and its potential vulnerability to impact by a released microorganism, is the soil and sediment detritus subsystem. First, the dynamics of this subsystem determine to a large extent the fertility of the autotrophs and thus the productivity of the remainder of the system. Second, the diversity of this system appears to be low, at least with respect to the microorganisms directly involved in transformations such as methane production, sulfate reduction, and denitrification. Low diversity suggests a subsystem extremely vulnerable to the appearance of competing microorganisms that could produce products that would violently disrupt the existing system. Third, although we know enough to say that the detritus substrate system is important, we do not really know very much about these systems as they exist in nature. For most such systems, it would be difficult to gather enough information to carry the structural analysis much beyond the crude example used for discussion in this chapter (Fig. 7.2). We already know that competition among microorganisms for organic substrates can produce rapid and large shifts in these processes, for example, in methane production versus sulfate reduction. Similar examples could arise through the accidental introduction of new forms with much more damaging consequences because of the lack of evolutionary time for stabilizing responses on the part of other populations. Processes such as lignin degradation, cellulose decomposition, and denitrification are all classed as important and vulnerable under any ecosystem structural analysis of the kind described in this chapter.

Information Flows and Functional Mechanisms of Control/Regulation

There is much less knowledge of flows of information and their incorporation into control mechanisms in ecosystems than of structural components and matter and energy flows (food webs). Prior to the advent of modeling as a tool of ecological research and the concurrent (but probably independent) rise of experimental field ecology and hypothesis testing, the need for such information was not perceived. There is, in fact, a rather large amount of useful information in the literature on life histories and on physiological ecology, but the observations and laboratory experiments are seldom designed to answer precisely the kind of questions raised by ecosystem structural and functional analyses.

Thus, since the methods discussed in this chapter depend at least initially on obtaining prior information about the system, in that respect they are presently inadequate.

CONCLUSIONS

Suitability of Structural Analysis

The methods of structural analysis outlined in this chapter, when strengthened by suitable information gathered about the ecosystem at risk and combined with data on the functional attributes of the system organisms, are appropriate for any ecosystem. Ideally, a combination of structural and functional analyses would produce a valid mechanistic model that would represent a synthesis of all that was known about the system. Additionally, such a model would have the capability of simulating the behavior of the system under a variety of proposed impacts and thus generate further testable conclusions. In general, in this model the bioengineered organisms appear as a separate compartment. This requirement can be made easier if one can discern subsystems within the target ecosystem that are relatively decoupled from each other, thus permitting specification on a much smaller and simpler scale. This is often possible with the soil detritus subsystem, for example. However, there is seldom the time, money, or opportunity to assemble and work with such a complete description. Thus, risk analysis must begin with component specification. Once the structural analysis is completed, however, different scenarios can be evaluated even in the complete absence of experimental data on control functions and parameter values. A model constructed entirely with parameter values taken from the literature at least can provide some sense of system vulnerability and parameter sensitivity, thus reducing the labor necessary to provide a sound mechanistic model. Depending on the importance of the particular system and on the immediacy and potential level of the risk, information gathering and analysis can proceed until the equilibrium between resources and risk is reached.

Needed Research

Some vital areas of ecological research must be designated if future capability for ecosystem risk analysis via structural (and functional) description is to improve. These include:

- Theoretical development based on ecological fact that emphasizes how observed or predicted properties of ecosystems arise through the interaction of structure with the functional attributes of components. Specifically, a small subset of control theories derived from the total number of species interactions found in any real ecosystem must be developed. At the same time, we need better exploration of systems theory aimed at explaining the relationships of small ecosystems integrated into larger, interacting sets of ecosystems at the regional and continental level.
- Experimental tests of theory by means of microcosms and mesocosms, and field plots, for example. Immediate attention should be given to microbially dominated ecosystem processes as well as the effects of these organisms and processes on other aspects of ecosystem behavior. Particular care should be taken to study the genotype variability within these microbial groups in order to estimate vulnerability to perturbations.
- Continuance of the multidisciplinary studies represented currently by the long-term ecological research sites, plus some additional long-term studies. If possible, the LTER program should be expanded to include a wider variety of sites, but in particular it should begin to replicate the same type of system at sites with recognizable differences in the expres-

sion of the ecosystem. If for each of the often useless impact studies an equal amount of money were set aside for basic descriptive or experimental research on a similar ecosystem, we could in the space of a decade or two really make some inroads into our current "data gap."

• Greatly expanded funding for taxonomic work and revisions in groups such as arthropods, other invertebrates, and microorganisms in soil and litter, where there are probably more new species than already have been described. Without research centers with competent individuals to provide identification, ecosystem analyses of the type described here cannot proceed.

REFERENCES

1. Christian, R. R. and R. L. Wetzel. 1978. Interactions between substrate microbes and consumers of *Spartina* "detritus" in estuaries. In M. Wiley (Ed.), *Estuarine Interactions*. Academic Press, New York, pp. 93–114.

2. Gardner, M. R. and W. R. Ashby. 1970. Connectance of large, dynamical (cybernetic) systems: Critical values for stability. *Nature* 228:784.

3. Hill, J. IV, and R. G. Wiegert. 1980. Microcosms in ecological modeling. In J. P. Giesy (Ed.), *Microcosms in Ecological Research*. Department of Energy Symposium Series 52, CONF-781101. U.S. Technical Information Center, Augusta, Ga., November 8–9, 1978.

4. May, R. M. 1973. *Stability and Complexity in Model Ecosystems*. Princeton University Press, Princeton, N.J.

5. Odum, E. P. 1971. *Fundamentals of Ecology*. 3rd ed. W. B. Saunders Co., Philadelphia

6. Odum, H. T. 1983. *Systems Ecology: An Introduction*. John Wiley and Sons, New York.

7. Smith, F. E. 1969. Effects of enrichment in mathematical models. In *Eutrophication*. National Academy of Sciences, Washington, D.C., pp. 631–645.

8. Smith, F. E. 1972. Spatial heterogeneity, stability, and diversity in ecosystems. *Trans. Conn. Acad. Arts & Sci.* 44:307–335.

9. Ulanowicz, R. 1980. An hypothesis on the development of natural communities. *J. Theor. Biol.* 85:223–245.

10. Wiegert, R. G., R. R. Christian, J. L. Gallagher, J. R. Hall, R. D. H. Jones, and R. L. Wetzel. 1975. A preliminary ecosystem model of a coastal Georgia *Spartina* marsh. In L. Eugene Cronin, *Estuarine Research. Chemistry, Biology and the Estuarine System*. Vol. 1. Academic Press, New York, pp. 583–601.

11. Wiegert, R. G., R. L. Wetzel, and R. R. Christian. 1981. A model view of the marsh. In L. Pomeroy and R. Wiegert (Eds.), *The Ecology of a Salt Marsh*. Springer Verlag, New York, pp. 183–218.

8

Controlled Testing and Monitoring Methods for Microorganisms

Gilbert S. Omenn

Evaluation of potential risks from deliberate release of genetically engineered organisms into the environment requires systematic, stepwise gathering of relevant empirical data. Speculating about and modeling potential risks will not suffice; a growing data base is essential for informed speculation about potential risks that need to be investigated and for modeling the survival, proliferation, function, and transport of introduced organisms and the expression and transfer of their genomes. Such a data base will be complementary to structural analysis prepared by others (see chapter 7, this volume).

The experience of the National Institutes of Health during the past decade with orderly development of risk assessment experiments provides a sound analogy for the broader questions that have been raised as this work moves beyond the controlled laboratory setting and industrial fermentation to field applications in agriculture, forestry, and pollution control [1,2]. The special attraction of recombinant DNA technology, and probably its inherent safety feature, is its specificity. Gene splicing can involve just one or very few specific genes for a specific purpose, contrasted with crossing the entire genome of two plants or fused protoplasts, for example. Genetic engineering strategies already employed include plasmid-mediated transfer of genes between bacteria or from Agrobacteria (*A. tumefaciens* or *A. rhizogenes*) to plants, deletion of specific genes for undesired functions, and transposition-mediated gene transfer. Obviously, success depends upon knowing the genes responsible for biologically significant functions; being able to isolate, clone, and introduce the gene into the desired recipient; having means to grow recipient cells into full plants or effective microbes; and being certain that the function of the introduced gene can be regulated as desired without negative effects on the recipient or the ecosystem in which it is expected to function.

It is certain that the applications of recombinant DNA techniques will be feasible sooner from manipulations of the microorganisms important in agriculture and in pollution control than for modification of traits for growth, habitat adaptation, resistance to environmental stressors, photosynthesis, or nitrogen fixation in plant species themselves. Microorganisms must be found or modified to meet demanding requirements of unusual environments, and they must survive and proliferate in competition with the existing flora, predators, and sometimes extreme or widely fluctuating chemical and physical conditions. The most promising prospects in environmental pollution control efforts relate genetically engineered organisms directly to manufacturing process modifications that have simple, consistent, and concentrated waste streams at the point of generation. Biochemical capacities in nature most likely to be useful are dehalogenation, deamination, denitration, and ring cleavage. Even partial detoxification of compounds already identified as hazardous under toxic waste and clean water regulations would be a useful step in overall disposal strategies. Lists of regulated chemicals may be considered directories of opportunity for genetic engineering. Similarly enhanced in situ degradation may be useful for toxic hot spots in sediments, soils, or sumps.

This very brief introduction about the opportunities for genetically engineered microorganisms in agriculture and pollution control provides the background for crucial recommendations that surely can reduce the likelihood of risk to the environment:

- Maximal information about the recipient and donor organisms utilized.
- High specificity and precision in the genetic change introduced.
- Use of recipient organisms well adapted to the habitat in which they are to be employed, with expression of their newly endowed specific attributes.
- Means of identifying and enumerating a reintroduced organism in the ecosystem.
- Means of monitoring its fate, including persistence, proliferation, and dispersion.

Methods must be developed for detection and enumeration of the introduced organism; detailed description of the patterns of release and spread of the organism; detection of gene transfer to and from other organisms; orderly recognition of toxicity, both acute and chronic, for nontarget species of many kinds; and detection of disruption of biogeochemical environmental processes. In every case, specific organisms, sites, and applications will be involved. It is no surprise that the Environmental Protection Agency and the National Institutes of Health have called for case-by-case assessments [3–5]. Nevertheless, certain methodologies are at the base of this field.

It is the purpose of this chapter to evaluate the suitability of empirical methods for assessing potential outcomes of environmental release of genetically modified organisms and to identify strengths, limitations, and research needs in these subfields that must be brought together.

METHODS FOR THE DETECTION, IDENTIFICATION, AND ENUMERATION OF NOVEL ORGANISMS

Sampling

Strategies for sampling depend upon the purpose, as noted recently by Glaser et al. [6] for an Environmental Protection Agency report on biotechnology [7]. To ascertain whether an introduced organism has persisted and carried out its desired functions, one must know the density and activity of the organism in the target field; thus, sampling must be intensive, local, and quantitative.

To cast a wide net over potential problems from transport beyond the site of application, it is necessary to sample a larger geographic area with methods that qualitatively identify the organism or its special genome and provide clues to the partitioning of the organism in various potential habitats or microhabitats. Sampling should include tissues and excreta from potential animal hosts. For our purposes, a combination of these approaches will be necessary.

Sediments and soils present problems for sampling because of the adsorption of microorganisms to various surfaces, from which desorption is unpredictable. Cells can be dissociated from solid phases by physical or chemical means and then be subjected to selective plate counting. Alternatively, the sediment or soil itself can be placed into broth enrichment medium, using replicated enrichments and replicated isolations from each flask. In either approach, molecular analyses can be grafted onto the culture method. The second approach is quite likely to detect genetically engineered microorganisms at lower densities than is possible with direct plate counting, and it is compatible with quantitation using most-probable-number (MPN) methods [7]. Designing an economical, but sufficient sampling strategy is a general problem in ecology; a performance curve of density against sampling effort can be a useful guide. Standard sources of information about sampling methods include those by Atlas and Bartha [8], Lynch and Poole [9], Sieburth [10], and Bergan [11].

Microbiological Culture Methods
with Marker Genes

Specific, convenient, reliable, and sensitive tracer methodologies are a prerequisite for the entire process of risk assessment in this field [12]. Microbiologists have relied upon the principles of selective enrichment or enhancement culture and differential media for nearly 100 years for the recovery and typing of organisms from various ecosystems. Various media are available for detection and differentiation of organisms according to their natural characteristics, especially metabolic requirements. The use of strains that are tagged with a particular metabolic activity or resistance attribute greatly facilitates the identification and enumeration of organisms of interest. For example, lactose fermentation might be a useful marker gene for bacteria other than *E. coli* (which is unusual in metabolizing lactose). Coliform-counting techniques could be used on M-Endo agar containing lactose and dyes that inhibit gram-positive bacteria; the agar turns metabolic green when lactose is metabolized to acidic products. To make a marker gene more specific, a convenient inducible promoter-operator sequence can be used. The tryptophan promoter-operator region would require presence of tryptophan for expression, and the phage lambda right operator could require high temperature or UV-irradiation for induction of the marker trait, whether lactose fermentation or some other trait is used.

Markers may be introduced conveniently on plasmids. For example, Masui et al. [13] described a plasmid in *E. coli* that induces production of the red-colored pigment prodigiosin. Application of a chemical or change of temperature may trigger induction of such chromogenic substances, an inexpensive and rapid means of identifying novel organisms. Obviously, if the plasmid is unstable and the DNA sequence of interest is not also carried on the plasmid, the marker will be unreliable.

There are limitations in the genetic markers available. The most convenient markers often are expressed as resistance to particular antibiotics, which suppress susceptible organisms, while the organism of interest may grow up from a very small initial proportion. After consulting with several leading microbiologists, Lindow and Panopoulos [14] reported the following list of candidates for resistance markers: novobiocin, aristocitin, hygromycin B, kasugamycin, bacitracin, fusidic acid, pimaricin, virginiamycin, nalidixic acid, bambermycin, tylomycin, and oleandromycin, plus heavy metals (e.g., Hg, Cd) [14]. It is essential to choose antibiotics that are not in use in humans or animals, since resistance to clinically useful antibiotics is a major public health problem. It is also important to use resistance genes that are located in the chromosome, not carried on easily transmissible extrachromosomal plasmids, and preferably not located in close proximity to repeated sequences which may function with transposable elements, in order to avoid extensive interspecies transfer. Some strains resistant to an antibiotic or a heavy metal ion do not grow well in the absence of that selective agent. Also, certain pesticides may interfere with heavy metal markers by inducing resistance among indigenous organisms. Finally, it is desirable to have at least two markers, so that a spontaneous mutation will not lead to disappearance of the singly tagged organism from the detection system.

Immunological Methods

Immunofluorescence techniques have been applied in microbial ecology for strains of Rhizobium species, Azotobacter, Beijerinckia, Azospirillium, nitrifiers, sulfur oxidizers, iron oxidizers, fungi, and other organisms [6]. However, there are several limitations to this approach. First, minimal countable densities in soils are 10^6 to 10^7 organisms/gm soil [15], depending upon desorption. This is too insensitive for our purposes. Second, other particles in the environment may fluoresce: inorganic particles may bind nonspecifically to the fluorescent antibody; certain materials autofluoresce; and there may be truly cross-reacting surface proteins on other organisms, or cross-reactions with contaminants present in the material in which the antiserum was produced. Third, the genetically engineered microorganism may not fluoresce due to organic slimes, as in the case of a fixed-bed wastewater treatment reactor [16], or because its antigen is not stable. Finally, immunofluorescence may not distinguish between living and dead cells and will not track the recombinant DNA gene itself, unless the antigen is specified by that DNA sequence.

Use of monoclonal antibodies offers substantial improvements in specificity, though not necessarily in sensitivity. Autofluorescence, interference by bacterial slimes, and inability to distinguish living and dead cells remain problems.

Genetic Analyses: Restriction Enzyme Mapping and Sequencing

Restriction enzymes, which specifically cleave DNA into easily separated and recognizable fragments, can be quite helpful in identifying and monitoring recombinant organisms. These naturally occurring enzymes have been the backbone of recombinant DNA advances in recent years; they cleave double-stranded DNA at specific sites determined by nucleotide sequences of four or six base pairs. Depending on the presence and location of the specific sequences, each restriction enzyme will yield a number of distinct fragments that can be separated according to their size on agarose gel electrophoresis. This approach is simplest with plasmids (limited amount of DNA). Restriction fragment patterns must be determined both for the nonrecombinant and recombinant plasmids (or chromosomal DNA). Inserted and deleted DNA would be identified through the changes in size of particular DNA fragments. Restriction enzymes are numerous and relatively expensive. It may be presumed that the manufacturer will be expected or required to perform the initial analyses of the sequences, ascertaining which enzyme (or enzymes) would be best for subsequent monitoring needs.

Restriction enzymes also represent a critical step toward sequencing genomes or plasmids. Church and Gilbert [17] have combined chemical sequencing of DNA [18] and Southern blotting [19] into a rapid method for sequencing regions of chromosomes direct from whole genomic DNA. Its applications in the near term will be limited to very special characterizations of fine structure. Another target for nucleotide sequencing, however, may be useful sooner, namely, the 5S ribosomal RNA. Several studies of *Vibrio cholerae* strains from marine environments have utilized sequencing methods to compare organisms from different sites or time periods or from the same environment with a notable difference in function [20,21]. Procaryotic 5S rRNA sequences between species vary by 5 to 15%, and within species a range of variation of about 2% has been found [20]. Thus, restriction mapping, probe hybridization (see below), and sequencing may be applied to 5S rRNA to identify organisms carrying gene markers, possibly in conjunction with probe analysis for the recombinant gene. There should be numerous situations in which it will be necessary to ascertain whether the gene of interest has been incorporated into additional species; rRNA analysis may become an efficient molecular means for showing that the gene has been transferred to a strain or species other than the one deliberately introduced.

Genetic Analyses: DNA Probes

When the specific DNA sequence is prepared for insertion into a recipient organism, a probe sequence complementary to the introduced sequence can be constructed for use in future monitoring efforts. The probe can be labeled for radioactive or fluorescent readout and can be hybridized to colonies growing on the surface of a nitrocellulose filter in contact with an appropriate medium. This technique is relatively expensive, and it depends upon adequate colony growth. Probe techniques do not enhance selective growth, nor do they provide a selective differential medium. Thus, traditional culture techniques must be coupled with the specificity of probe hybridization.

The most popular substitute for ^{32}P-radioactive labeling is the fluorescent method based upon the biotin/avidin high-affinity complex [22,23]. A great variety of readout technologies is under development.

The length and sequence of the probe depend upon the host-vector system that is utilized. When the recombinant DNA is an altered gene that normally is present in that host, the differences in sequence may be as small as a single nucleotide, so that very carefully defined hybridization conditions will be necessary to demonstrate the difference. In contrast, the methodology is much simpler when a wholly new gene is introduced.

The colony hybridization method [24] currently has sensitivity capable of detecting one colony in 10^6 of a nonhomologous DNA background [25]. Amplification methods for labeled probes tied to fluorescent or luminescent or colorimetric products of enzyme cascades likely will increase the sensitivity by two orders of magnitude or more [C. R. Burke, Allied Health and Scientific Products, personal communication, 1984].

Probe analysis can be combined with the restriction enzyme mapping described above to test whether the organism isolated from the environment, compared with the restriction fragment pattern for the original recombinant organism, still has the recombinant sequence in the original position, and whether it has undergone any detectable alterations or deletions. The method may be unable to detect point mutations or certain inversions. Additional tests, using monoclonal antibodies for detecting metabolic or resistance properties, are necessary to ascertain that the recombinant gene actually is producing its gene product.

METHODS FOR ASSESSING FATE AND EFFECTS OF GENETICALLY ENGINEERED ORGANISMS

In striking contrast with the situation of organisms that may be released accidentally to the environment from laboratory or industrial applications, organisms released deliberately to function in the environment must be able to survive, proliferate, and express their desired functions. Many microbial ecologists have emphasized what an enormous challenge it will be to introduce truly novel organisms into well adapted habitats [2,26]. This caution applies not only to microbes, but also to plant and animal species [2, p. 178]. Nevertheless, some troubling examples are known of invading organisms that became pests or strikingly changed a particular habitat. Chestnut blight due to a parasitic Asian fungus, *Endothia parasitica*; the Gypsy moth, *Lymantria dispar*; the mongoose, *Herpestes auropunctates*; kudzu; and the Japanese beetle [27,28] are classic examples. Insects introduced as counterparts have been both successes and problems, the latter usually reflecting undesirably broad host range. There should be lessons that can be applied from these unusual negative experiences; most important, that broad host range is undesirable.

Empirical assessment of the fate, transport, gene transfer, and ecosystem effects of introduced organisms should begin with totally contained systems that simulate terrestrial or aquatic environments of interest. These environments range from flasks, mason jars, and growth chambers on the laboratory bench to fully contained greenhouses and systematically sampled natural areas, sometimes termed mesocosms. There are two types of microcosms [29–31]. The first is naturally derived. A sample of soil, lake water, or marine sediment may be brought into the laboratory for analysis. The naturally derived microcosm represents an excised natural community. The second type of microcosm is synthesized or standardized with chemically defined media. Indicator organisms must be chosen and introduced to make a biologically meaningful and ecologically instructive multitrophic system.

Naturally Derived Microcosms

The Environmental Protection Agency has developed programs for both terrestrial and aquatic research [12]. The approach builds upon several decades of studies on the persistence of certain microorganisms in natural ecosystems, especially organisms associated with animals and plants as pathogens or pollution-indicator bacteria. More contemporary information needs to be gained about persistence, cell densities, and fate of species such as *Pseudomonas*, *Xanthomonas*, *Erwinia* and *Klebsiella*, which are associated with the plant phyllosphere and root rhizosphere, and about *Pseudomonas*, *Vibrio*, *Nitrosomonas*, *Alcaligenes*, *Actineobacter*, *Aeromonas*, and others found in fresh and marine water systems.

The terrestrial model that the Environmental Protection Agency is developing will be used to investigate the following five ecosystems: rhizobium/legume/soil, root rhizosphere of easily manipulated and cultivated plants (radishes and potatoes), soil/plant systems for investigating fate and effects of engineered organisms capable of biodegrading certain pesticides, vegetables undergoing microbial decay, and plant leaf surfaces [12]. Natural terrestrial habitats have been selected that support high natural cell density. For example, an average legume nodule contains 10^7 to 10^9 viable cells [32] and plant root rhizospheres contain 10^6 or more bacteria per cm length of root surface [33]. The spray application of herbicide-degrading bacteria onto soil and plants will probably not achieve high cell densities, unless there is a significant regrowth of the organism. However, many of the indigenous soil bacteria may be killed by the herbicide, making both nutrients and niches available for the resistant engineered or selected plasmid-containing microbe. The natural decay of vegetation in the pesticide model and in the post-harvest vegetable leaf-decay model will lead to marked changes in terrestrial microflora, especially plant-pathogenic soft-rot bacteria of the genera *Erwinia*, *Pectobacterium*, and *Pseudomonas*.

Since these organisms undergo promiscuous plasmid transfer [2,34–36], they are ideal for following the fate of well marked novel genomes.

Studies with naturally derived aquatic systems may utilize ecocores taken from the sediment of lakes, streams, and estuaries. Bourquin and Pritchard of the Environmental Protection Agency have used such ecocores to determine degradation rates of xenobiotics by the organisms present in the sediments [2,37]. Ecosystems with high microbial densities are most likely to foster gene flow between species components; these include certain aquatic sediments, salt marsh sediments, and various liquid to surface interfaces.

Cell-to-cell movement of genes is thought to depend more on ecological intimacy than on evolutionary relatedness [37]. Such a conclusion can be investigated in aquatic microcosms, admittedly with many simplifying assumptions.

Grimes, Singleton, and Colwell [38] have reported an instructive use of microcosms to investigate a hypothesis based upon observations in the natural marine environment. The Puerto Rico Trench surface water of the Atlantic Ocean was the dump site for some 3.6×10^8 liters of composite pharmaceutical waste (CPW) per year from 1972 through 1981. Contrary to expectations, the culturable bacterial community in the dump site was dominated by *Vibrio* species rather than by *Pseudomonas* [39]. It was hypothesized that the pharmaceutical wastes had led to a restructuring of the culturable heterotrophic bacterial community. To test this allogenic succession hypothesis, laboratory experiments were conducted. The culturable bacterial flora of Chesapeake Bay water samples, when treated with CPW, showed not only no apparent toxic effects, but also an increase in number of bacteria. Next, microcosms containing two species communities (*Vibrio* PR-110 and *Pseudomonas* AO-17 or AO-66) were studied, and *Vibrio* both was dominant and increased its dominance in relation to dose of wastes added. Obviously, it is a long way from recognizing these shifts in marine bacterial communities to understanding the direct and indirect consequences on the overall ecosystem.

Synthesized or Standardized Microcosms

Taub and her colleagues at the University of Washington, with support from the Food and Drug Administration over the past decade, have developed experimental microcosms with chemically defined media and a variety of algae, grazers, and detritivores [40–43]. These synthetic microcosms are composed of distilled water, silica sand, reagent-grade chemicals, and organisms that are easily reared in the laboratory. The species presently included in these microcosms are listed in Table 8.1.

These systems provide a non-site-specific, ecosystem-level bioassay with

Table 8.1. Standardized Aquatic Microcosm

Algae		Animals	
Anabaena	Blue-greens	Daphnia magna	
Ankistrodesmus	Large greens	Cyprinotus vidua	Ostracod
Chlamydomonas	Small greens	Hyalella	Amphipod
Chlorella	Small greens	Philodina	Rotifers
Nitzschia kutzInglana	Diatoms	Hypotrichs	Protozoans
Lyngbya	Blue-greens		
Scenedesmus	Colonial greens		
Selenastrum	Small greens		
Stigeoclonium	Filamentous greens		
Ulothrix	Filamentous greens		

Note: The rationale for choices of these species is presented in Taub and Crow [40].

interspecies competition within primary, secondary, and recycling trophic levels. Thirty or 60 replicate microcosms in 3-liter bottles can be set up to allow manipulation of physical and chemical variables of interest, dose-response studies, and reproducibility of observations. The microcosms display nutrient depletion, algal competition and succession, and algal depletion through grazing and nutrient depletion. External agents can be assayed in different phases of maturation of these synthesized ecosystems [41].

For example, the antibiotic streptomycin acted as a selective algal toxicant, markedly reducing all indices of primary production (carbon uptake, extracted chlorophyll, in vivo fluorescence, cell abundance, and pH) during the first two weeks. Its effects were manifested as modified algal dominance relationships over the 63-day experiment. Although no active drug could be detected by day 28, late effects included reduced Daphnia populations and markedly increased ostracod populations. Another set of experiments using the pesticide malathion showed a temporary reduction in the number of grazers with a concurrent algal bloom. Degradation of the malathion was not measured; however, it could be presumed to occur as the grazer populations recovered. Their recovery was accompanied by elimination of the algal bloom [42]. In contrast, at the same concentration, malathion was slightly stimulatory to some algae and highly toxic to ostracods, amphipods, and Daphnia in single species bioassays. Thus, these microcosms represent a significant step toward revealing complexity in ecosystem responses and effects.

A variety of measurements and observations can be made over the course of an extensive protocol in the microcosm, and recovery from temporary toxicities can be demonstrated because of the periodic (usually weekly) reinoculation of small numbers of organisms. Considerable sophistication in data management has been achieved, but more extensive biochemical measurements need to be developed. The operational costs are low, with all the supplies readily available through chemical and scientific supply companies. All of the master solutions are stable and can be stored for long periods of time. In addition, the organism cultures are available through multiple sources and have been highly standardized. The Food and Drug Administration currently is supporting an interlaboratory testing protocol that involves the University of Washington, the Aberdeen Laboratories of the Army, the Duluth Laboratory of the Environmental Protection Agency, and the laboratories of a private consulting company. The test agent under study is copper sulfate, which is commonly used as an algicide in reservoirs to maintain water quality.

Swartzman and Rose have presented a strategy for improved prediction of the biological effects of toxicant additions to aquatic microcosms. The approach involves combining single-species bioassay results with microcosm and mesocosm studies, using simulation models to predict the nutrient-cycle responses of natural ecosystems and the likely toxic effects on phytoplankton and zooplankton [44]. Their scheme is outlined in Figure 8.1.

To introduce microorganisms instead of chemicals in these systems, the sampling techniques would have to be altered extensively to prevent escape of the test organisms and to assure aseptic technique. Large organisms would have to be sampled without removal, and resultant counts would be approximate. Microscopic counts would have to be handled quite differently. Scraping of wall surfaces presumably could be managed externally with magnetic control of internal scrapers. Even so, the Food and Drug Administration clearly expects this system to be useful for microorganism testing [45].

Biological pest control agents include viruses as well as bacteria. The nuclear polyhedrosis viruses (baculoviruses) are particularly of interest. A report has appeared testing this virus, isolated from the Alfalfa looper, *Autographa californica*, on the grass shrimp, *Palaemonetes vulgaris*, as a nontarget aquatic species. Histopathological, ultrastructural, and serological methods provided no evidence of infection or pathogenicity [46].

Mesocosms

Well-controlled environments outside the laboratory are a critical step before open field trials. The greenhouse and the controlled field site are well-established tools of biologists for planting and observing species of

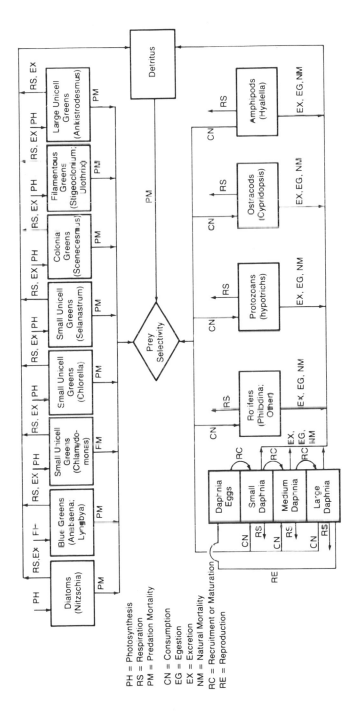

PH = Photosynthesis
RS = Respiration
PM = Predation Mortality

CN = Consumption
EG = Egestion
EX = Excretion
NM = Natural Mortality
RC = Recruitment or Maturation
RE = Reproduction

Figure 8.1. Biomass flows in a phytoplankton-zooplankton simulation model. Flows involving the recycling of nitrogen and phosphorus through the detrital compartment are not shown. (From Swartzman and Rose [44], with permission.)

155

interest, as well as their responses to microbial and chemical sprays, irrigation schemes, and other manipulations. For aquatic environments, flow-through systems with bags or tanks are often utilized; however, these are not closed environments.

With regard to microbial agents, the extensive much debated record on ice nucleation mutants of *Pseudomonas syringae* and *Erwinia herbiocola* is the best available example. The submission to the National Institutes of Health includes studies of bean plants and corn seedlings incubated in mist chambers in greenhouses, plus field studies of frost injury to immature Bartlett pear fruit and newly emerging potato leaves [47]. In recently reaffirming their approval for limited field studies, the National Institutes of Health were able to cite evidence about the biological and ecological characteristics of the nonmodified parental organisms, as well as the modified organism, and logically conclude that unintended agricultural and meteorological effects would be insignificant or nonexistent [47]. The mutant strains, when tested in a growth chamber and greenhouse environment, did not induce injury to plants and were not capable of colonizing leaves to a greater extent than the original strain. Studies of the behavior of bacteria colonizing leaf surfaces supported a strong case that the planned introduction of ice nucleation-negative, genetically engineered bacteria would be very unlikely to have a significant effect beyond local competition on the leaf surface with ice nucleation-positive bacterial relatives. Naturally occurring and chemically induced ice nucleation-negative mutants already have been studied in the field, since no restrictions apply to these analogues of the genetically engineered mutant.

Survival, lateral dissemination, and population dynamics of nucleation-negative mutants and nucleation-positive populations, and the specificity of their interactions on leaf surfaces, can be studied much better in controlled field sites than in greenhouses. The proposed field test will permit measurements of the applied bacteria at 10 meters, 100 meters, and 1,000 meters in all directions, utilizing antibiotic resistance and DNA sequence markers. As in the laboratory, the sensitivity of detection of effects depends on the measures to be employed. No biocides will be used to destroy the treated plants; all above-ground plant parts will be buried at the test site. As the proposed frost prevention experiments illustrate, specific biological and ecological monitoring must be designed case by case. The problem of frost damage at temperatures just a few degrees below freezing is a major worldwide agricultural challenge. Many dozens of species of agricultural and wild plants harbor epiphytic ice nucleation-active bacteria.

The expression of an introduced gene and its effects on the growth and survival of a plant should first be studied in the greenhouse. Examples under development include incorporation of the gene for *Bacillus thuringiensis* toxin, which might make tobacco or other plants resistant to

Lepidoptera larvae without chemical or bacterial sprays; incorporation of the gene for EPSP synthase for resistance of plants to glyphosate (Round-Up®) or other herbicides; and increasing the protein levels in forage crops, the quality of seed proteins, or the photosynthetic activity of plants (via genes for components of ribulose-1,5-bis phosphate carboxylase/oxylase). Manipulation of plants is limited at this point by the availability of effective vectors, the best of which appears to be the Ti plasmid derived from *Agrobacterium tumefaciens*. All of these manipulations are aimed at increasing crop yield, often through enhanced resistance to environmental stressors. Thus, these crop products may compare better in their normal environments. Without a selective advantage and active selective pressures, the introduction of new or altered genes may make either the microorganisms or plants less efficient and less competitive, especially if plasmids must be housed [35].

There are likely to be numerous indirect effects on other species via effects on available nutrients and other resources. Determination of what signal processes could be measured will have to be decided on a case-by-case basis, for the time being following the "Points to Consider" document of the Recombinant DNA Advisory Committee working group. It should be noted that many plant breeders feel confident that genetically engineered organisms will behave indistinguishably from strains improved genetically by crossbreeding and various plant tissue culture methods [28], but no detailed ecological studies have been done to substantiate these claims.

For pollution control applications, there should be an analogous scaling up from the laboratory to pilot simulations of waste treatment facilities, agricultural and forestry decomposition sites, contaminated soil sites, mineral leaching from ores, or oil sump cleanup sites. The ecocore approach seems well suited to bringing samples of these various target environmental applications into a fully contained environment, in which the desired microorganisms can be introduced and monitored for their fate and effects. The entire operation can be incinerated or sealed for disposal. As in the examples above, markers for following the organism and its genome and multiple measures of effects in the target environment must be built into case-specific protocols.

It should be emphasized that as toxic waste sites in the environment are sealed or removed, there are appropriate and varied opportunities for testing organisms with specific degradative capabilities, or mixed cultures of organisms with a variety of capabilities, in an effort to detoxify the more intractable and toxic agents in the site at least partially [2]. It should be possible to use a well-demarcated portion of the site and to monitor the fate and effects of the introduced organisms, always with the capacity to seal the operation as previously planned. Less controlled field sites represent an enormous array of site-specific needs, opportunities, and potential risks. There must be adequate assurance that the organisms have shown no cause for concern in microcosm studies, have highly specific properties, and preferably are drawn from a site to which they may be returned or a similar ecological habitat, and that decontamination of the entire operation is feasible. It is possible that organisms could be modified so as to "disarm" them ecologically, so they will not be likely to spread beyond the range where they are intended to be effective, or so that they can be "recalled" through sensitivity to certain antibiotics or bacterial phage [48]. We must take care, however, that the protection does not introduce greater hazards than the organism itself.

METHODS FOR ASSESSING GENETIC STABILITY OF GENETICALLY ENGINEERED ORGANISMS

Genetic stability studies must address some of the more speculative concerns about this work. It is conceivable that even a seemingly precise recombinant DNA experiment might carry along transcription signals or coding sequences that would have unpredicted effects in additional host organisms. Repeated sequences or transposons might lead to multiple and unintended insertions, with disruption or conceivably activation of certain host genes. Some of these speculations are difficult to operationalize, but it is possible systematically to look at the likelihood of transfer of DNA sequences between species. This is particularly true in cases when the inserted DNA sequences are carried on extrachromosomal plasmids, which are known to be readily transferred across species. An empirical approach is needed to address issues of host range, because theory is weak, both for gene transfer and for toxicity [49].

Organisms can initially be grown to high cell densities in laboratory media and combined with bacteria likely to be encountered in nature. Using routine selective media, such mixed cultures can be examined for recombinant organisms receiving the marker genes. Comparable studies can be carried out with naked DNA and with intact organisms to assess the stability of marker DNA sequences in plasmids and in chromosomal sites, also checking for transfer frequencies due to transformation or transduction or conjugation mechanisms. Since plasmid DNA is certain to be released from lysed bacterial cells, it is useful to inquire about the fate and effects resulting from release of plasmid DNA into specific niches such as legume root nodules, root rhizospheres, or pollutant degradation sites in water or soil systems [12].

Table 8.2 indicates the genera of bacteria likely to be exchanging broad host range plasmids in the respective ecosystems. Triparental matings may be essential to analyze as well. Helper plasmids in terrestrial microcosm flora and contributions of transposons should be searched for specifically. Here again, a combination of microcosms and effective marker attributes will permit studies of considerably higher complexity than two-species or even mixed-culture chemostat experiments. The combination is central to the stepwise, systematic, empirical investigation of these organisms.

We have powerful tools for developing this field. However, very few applications can be cited thus far with organisms of interest for agricultural or environmental applications. As noted, great care must be exercised in the choice of marker genes and phenotypes, to avoid introducing unnecessary risks from the monitoring process. In many situations, the growth of introduced organisms will be limited and the dilution by natural flora will be so great, that DNA probe or monoclonal antibody reagents will be useful only after successful selection and enrichment for the desired organism. Obviously, it will be even more difficult to use the same diagnostic tools to trace the genome into minor species in the environment. On the other hand, should gene transfer occur into an organism that becomes a dominant species, these diagnostic tools might be highly effective.

CONCLUSIONS

Molecular, microbiological, and ecological tools are already available for empirical studies that should steadily advance our knowledge and narrow our uncertainties about the effects of genetically engineered indigenous organisms. It will be much more difficult to anticipate the behavior and effects of nonindigenous organisms, whether genetically engineered or not.

Table 8.2. Genera To Be Investigated for Gene Transfer

Ecosystem	Genera
Soil	*Pseudomonas, Alcaligenes, Klebsiella, Enterobacter, Rhizobium*
Aquatic	*Pseudomonas, Escherichia, Klebsiella*
Marine	*Vibrio*
Plant-associated	*Pseudomonas, Alcaligenes, Agrobacterium, Citrobacter, Enterobacter, Erwinia Pectobacterium, Klebsiella*
Invertebrate and mammalian	*Escherichia coli* plus several genera listed above

From the Environmental Protection Agency [12], illustrative approach.

Despite the paucity of published papers in our literature search, the microcosm-greenhouse-mesocosm approach must be considered a promising strategy for future use. Examples with chemical toxicants in synthesized microcosms are encouraging. The investigation of actions of naturally occurring and introduced microorganisms in estuarine ecocores similarly can be expanded.

Nevertheless, the complexity of ecosystems is such that site-specific naturally derived communities and convenient multitrophic synthesized microcosms represent only snapshots in a dynamic panorama. Which site should be chosen, which species should be introduced, and what physical and chemical conditions should be tested all greatly influence the results. The challenge is to find sensitive and meaningful correlation in microcosms with the effects seen or not seen in greenhouses, in controlled field sites, and eventually in open field applications. It would be helpful if we knew more about the complex ecological responses to chemical pesticides and to the dozen EPA-approved nongenetically engineered microbial pesticides (of which the most used is *Bacillus thuringiensis* for control of the Gypsy moth) [3,50]. It is clear that such expansion of research and training in the many aspects of ecology in this area will be necessary in order to address these questions. It is not likely, however, that genetically engineered organisms, especially when drawn from the habitats into which they will be reintroduced, carry any greater risk than the agents with which we consider ourselves familiar.

In the meantime, models and speculations about risks from deliberate release of genetically engineered organisms are informed minimally by actual observations. As always, there is less confidence and higher estimates of risk when data are poor. This field can surely be advanced and the models much better informed if the lead agencies of the government, namely the Environmental Protection Agency and the Department of Agriculture, would carry out and stimulate orderly research and development on pollution control and agricultural needs. Such developmental work can be combined with the stepwise investigation of potential ecological effects, demonstrating for others how to advance the field responsibly.

REFERENCES

1. Levin, B. R. 1984. Changing views of the hazards of recombinant DNA manipulation and the regulation of these procedures. *Recombinant DNA Tech. Bull.* 7:107–114.
2. Omenn, G. S. and A. Hollaender. 1984. *Genetic Control of Environmental Pollutants.* Plenum Press, New York.
3. U.S. Environmental Protection Agency. 1984. Proposed policy regarding certain microbiol products. *Federal Register* 49:50880–50897.
4. Milewski, E. and S. A. Tolin. 1984. Development of guidelines for field test-

ing of plants modified by recombinant DNA techniques. *Recombinant DNA Tech. Bull.* 7:114–124.

5. National Institutes of Health (In preparation). Points to consider for submissions involving testing in the environment of microorganisms derived by recombinant DNA techniques.

6. Glaser, D., T. Keith, P. Riley, G. Chambers, J. Manning, S. Hattingh, and R. Evans. 1984. Monitoring techniques for genetically engineered microorganisms. Commissioned report of Environmental Protection Agency Biotechnology Workshop. Environmental Protection Agency, Washington, D.C.

7. Russek, E. and R. R. Colwell. 1983. Computation of most probable numbers. *Appl. Environ. Microbiol* 45.1646–1650.

8. Atlas, R. M. and R. Bartha. 1981. *Microbial Ecology: Fundamentals and Applications.* Addison-Wesley, Reading, Mass.

9. Lynch, J. M. and N. J. Poole, Eds. 1979. *Microbial Ecology: A Conceptual Approach.* Blackwell Scientific Publications, Oxford.

10. Sieburth, J. M. 1979. *Sea Microbes.* Oxford University Press, New York.

11. Bergan, T. 19xx. Human- and animal-pathogenic members of the genus *Pseudomonas.* In M. P. Starr, et al. (Eds.), *The Procaryotes.* Springer-Verlag, New York.

12. U.S. Environmental Protection Agency. 1984. Biotechnology Workshop, draft paper. Office of Environmental Processes and Effects Research, Coolfont, W. Va.

13. Masui, Y., T. Mizuno, and M. Inouye. 1984. Novel high-level expression cloning vehicles: 10^4-fold amplification of *Escherichia coli* minor protein. *Biotech.* 2:81–85.

14. Lindow, S. E. and N. J. Panopoulos. 1983. Request for permission to test *P. syringae* pv. *syringae* and *Erwinia herbicola* carrying specific deletions in ice nucleation genes under field conditions as biocontrol agents of frost injury to plants. Revised protocol for Recombinant DNA Committee, National Institutes of Health, Washington, D.C.

15. Bohlool, B. B. and E. F. Schmidt. 1980. The immunofluorescence approach in mocrobial ecology. *Adv. Microb. Ecol.* 4:203–242.

16. Szwerinski, H., S. Gaiser, and D. Bardtke. 1985. Immunofluorescence for the quantitative determination of nitrifying bacteria interference of the test in biofilm reactors. *Appl. Microbiol. Biotechnol.* 21:125–128.

17. Church, G. M. and W. Gilbert. 1984. Genomic sequencing. *Proc. Natl. Acad. Sci. U.S.A.* 81:1991–1995.

18. Maxam, A. M. and W. Gilbert. 1980. Sequencing end-labeled DNA with base-specific chemical cleavages. *Meth. Enzymol.* 65:499–560.

19. Southern, E. M. 1975. Detection of specific sequences among DNA fragments separated by gel electrophoresis. *J. Mol. Biol.* 98:503–517.

20. MacDonell, M. T. and R. R. Colwell. 1984. Identical 5S rRNA nucleotide sequence of *Vibrio cholerae* strains representing temporal, geographical, and ecological diversity. *Appl. Environ. Microbiol.* 48:119–121.

21. Deming, J. W., R. Hada, R. R. Colwell, K. R. Luehrsen, and G. E. Fox. 1984. The ribonucleotide sequence of 5S rRNA from two strains of deep-sea barophilic bacteria. *J. Gen. Microbiol.* 130:1911–1920.

22. Langer, P. R., A. A. Waldrop, and D. O. Ward. 1981. Enzymatic synthesis of biotin-labeled polynucleotides: Novel nucleic acid affinity probes. *Proc. Natl. Acad. Sci. U.S.A.* 78:6633–6637.

23. Lewin, R. 1983. Genetic probes become ever sharper. *Science* 221:1167.

24. Grunstein, M. and D. S. Hogness. 1975. Colony hybridization: A method for

the isolation of cloned DNAs that contain a specific gene. *Proc. Natl. Acad. Sci. U.S.A. 72*:3961–3965.

25. Sayler, G. S., M. S. Shields, E. T. Tedford, A. Breen, S. W. Hooper, K. M. Sirotkin, and J. W. Davis. 1985. Application of DNA-DNA colony hybridization to the detection of catabolic genotypes in environmental samples. *Appl. Environ. Microbiol. 49*:1295–1303.

26. Alexander, M. 1981. Why microbial predators and parasites do not eliminate their prey and hosts. *Ann. Rev. Microbiol. 35*:113–133.

ĸ 27. Sharples, F. E. 1983. Spread of organisms with novel genotypes: Thoughts from an ecological perspective. *Recombinant DNA Tech. Bull. 6*:43–56.

ṵ 28. Brill, W. J. 1985. Safety concerns and genetic engineering in agriculture. *Science 227*:381–384.

29. Gillet, J. W. and J. M. Witt, Eds. 1977. Terrestrial microcosms: Proceedings of a workshop. National Science Foundation, Washington, D.C.

30. Giesy, J. P., Jr., Ed. 1980. Microcosms in ecological research. Department of Energy Symposium, CONF-781101, Series 52, Washington, D.C.

31. Grice, G. D. and M. R. Reeve, Eds. 1982. *Marine Mesocosms: Biological and Chemical Research in Experimental Ecosystems.* Springer-Verlag, New York.

32. Kosslak, R. M., B. E. Bohlool, S. Dowdle, and M. J. Sardowsy. 1983. Competition of *Rhizobium meliloti* strains in early stages of soybean nodulation. *Appl. Environ. Microbiol. 46*:870–873.

33. Kloepper, J. W., M. N. Schroth, and T. D. Miller. 1980. Effects of rhizosphere colonization by plant growth-promoting rhizobacteria on potato plant development and yield. *Phytopathol. 70*:1078–1082.

34. Chakrabarty, A. M. 1976. Plasmids in Pseudomonas. *Ann. Rev. Genetics 10*:7–30.

•35. Stotsky, G. and H. Babich. Fate of genetically engineered microbes in natural environments. *Recombinant DNA Tech. Bull. 7*:163–188.

36. Stotsky, G. and V. N. Krasovky. 1981. Ecological factors that affect the survival, establishment, growth and genetic recombination of microbes in natural habitats. In B. S. Levy, C. Clowes, and E. L. Koenig (Eds.), *Molecular Biology, Pathogenicity, and Ecology of Bacterial Plasmids.* Plenum Press, New York, pp. 31–42.

37. Pritchard, P. H., A. W. Bourquin, H. L. Frederickson, and T. Maziarz. 1979. System design factors affecting environmental fate studies in microcosms. In A. W. Bourquin and P. H. Pritchard (Eds.), *Proceedings of the Workshop: Microbial Degradation of Pollutants in Marine Environments.* EPA-600/9-79-012, pp. 251–272.

38. Grimes, D. J., F. L. Singleton, and R. R. Colwell. 1984. Allogenic succession of marine bacterial communities in response to pharmaceutical waste. *J. Appl. Bacteriol. 57*:247–261.

39. Peele, E. R., F. L. Singleton, J. W. Deming, B. Cavari, and R. R. Colwell. 1981. Effects of pharmaceutical wastes on microbial populations in surface waters at the Puerto Rico dumpsite in the Atlantic Ocean. *Appl. Environ. Microbiol. 41*:873–879.

40. Taub, F. B. and M. E. Crow. 1980. Synthesizing aquatic microcosms. In J. P. Giesy, Jr. (Ed.), *Microcosms in Ecological Research.* Department of Energy Symposium, Series 52, pp. 69–104.

41. Kindig, A. C., L. L. Conquest, and F. B. Taub. 1983. Differential sensitivity of new versus mature synthetic microcosms to streptomycin sulfate treatment. In W. E. Bishop, R. D. Cardwell, and B. E. Heidolph (Eds.), *Aquatic*

Toxicology and Hazard Assessment: Sixth Symposium. American Society of Testing and Materials, Philadelphia, pp. 192–203.

42. Taub, P. E., P. L. Read, A. C. Kindig, M. C. Harrass, H. J. Hartmann, L. L. Conquest, F. J. Hardy, and P. T. Munro. 1983. Demonstrations of the ecological effects of streptomycin and malathion on synthetic aquatic microcosms. In W. E. Bishop, R. D. Cardwell, and B. B. Heidolph (Eds.), *Aquatic Toxicology and Hazard Assessment: Sixth Symposium.* American Society for Testing and Materials, Philadelphia, pp. 5–25.

43. Taub, F. B. 1984. Synthetic microcosms as biological models of algal communities. In L. E. Shubert (Ed.), *Algae as Ecological Indicators.* Academic Press, New York, pp. 363–394.

44. Swartzman, G. L. and K. A. Rose. 1983. Simulating the biological effects of toxicants in aquatic microcosm systems. *Ecol. Modeling* 22:123–134.

45. Chemical Regulation Reporter. 1984. Assessment of RDNA microbe survivability may be possible with microcosm ecosystem test. *Bureau of National Affairs,* November 23, pp. 978–979.

46. Couch, J. A., S. M. Martin, G. Tompkins, and J. Kinney. 1984. A simple system for the preliminary evaluation of infectivity and pathogenesis of insect virus in a nontarget estuarine shrimp *Palaemonetes vulgaris. J. Invertebr. Pathol.* 43:351–357.

47. Wyngaarden, J. B. 1985. Lindow and Panopoulos proposal concerning ice nucleation bacteria. Environmental assessment and finding of no significant impact. National Institutes of Health, January 21.

48. Brown, J. H., R. K. Colwell, R. E. Lenski, B. R. Levin, M. Lloyd, P. J. Regal, and D. Simberloff. 1984. Report on workshop on possible ecological and evolutionary impacts of bioengineered organisms released into the environment. *Bull. Ecol. Soc. Amer.* 65:436–438.

49. U.S. Congress, Subcommitttee on Investigations and Oversight. 1984. *The Environmental Implications of Genetic Engineering.* Staff Report.

50. U.S. Environmental Protection Agency. 1979. Policy statement on biorational pesticides. *Federal Register* 44:23994.

APPENDIX

Points to Consider for Submissions Involving Testing in the Environment of Microorganisms Derived by Recombinant DNA Techniques

Department of Health and Human Services, National Institutes of Health

Experiments in this category require specific review by the Recombinant DNA Advisory Committee (RAC) and approvals by the National Institutes of Health (NIH) and the Institutional Biosafety Committee (IBC) before initiation. The IBC is expected to make an independent evaluation, although this evaluation need not occur before consideration of an experiment by the RAC. Relevant information on the proposed experiments should be submitted to the Office of Recombinant DNA activities (ORDA). The objective of this review procedure is to evaluate the potential environmental effects of testing of microorganisms that have been modified by recombinant DNA techniques.

These following points to consider have been developed by the RAC Working Group on Release into the Environment as a suggested list for scientists preparing proposals on environmental testing of microorganisms, including viruses, that have been modified using recombinant DNA techniques. The review of proposals for environmental testing of modified organisms is being done on a case-by-case basis, because the range of possible organisms, applications, and environments indicates that no standard set of procedures is likely to be appropriate in all circumstances. However, some common considerations allow the construction of points such as those below.

Information on all these points will not be necessary in all cases but will depend on the properties of the parental organism and the effect of the modification on these properties.

From *Federal Register*, Part II, Vol. 50, No. 60, March 28, 1985.

Approval of small-scale field tests will depend upon the results of laboratory and greenhouse testing of the properties of the modified organism. We anticipate that monitoring of small-scale field tests will provide data on environmental effects of the modified organism. Such data may be a necessary part of the consideration of requests for approval of large-scale tests and commercial application.

I. Summary

Present a summary of the proposed trial, including objectives, significance, and justification for the request.

II. Genetic Considerations of Modified Organism to be Tested

A. Characteristics of the Nonmodified Parental Organism

1. Information on identification, taxonomy, source, and strain.
2. Information on the organism's reproductive cycle and capacity for genetic transfer.

B. Molecular Biology of the Modified Organism

1. Introduced Genes
   a. Source and function of the DNA sequence used to modify the organism to be tested in the environment.
   b. Identification, taxonomy, source, and strain on organisms donating the DNA.
2. Construction of the Modified Organism
   a. Describe the method(s) by which the vector with insert(s) has been constructed. Include diagrams as appropriate.
   b. Describe the method of introduction of the vector carrying the insert into the organism to be modified and the procedure for selection of the modified organism.
   c. Specify the amount and nature of any vector or donor DNA remaining in the modified organism.
   d. Give the laboratory containment conditions specified by the NIH guidelines for the modified organisms.
3. Genetic Stability and Expression
   a. Present results and interpretation of preliminary tests designed to measure genetic stability and expression of the introduced DNA in the modified organism.

III. Environmental Considerations

The intent of gathering ecological information is to assess the effects of survival, reproduction, and/or dispersal of the modified organism. For this purpose, information should be provided where possible and appropriate on relevant ecological characteristics of the nonmodified organism, the corresponding characteristics of the modified organism, and the physiological and ecological role of donated genetic sequences in the donor and in the modified organism. For the following points, provide information where possible and appropriate on the nonmodified organism, and a prediction of any change that may be elicited by the modification.

A. Habitat and Geographic Distribution
B. Physical and Chemical Factor(s) That Can Affect Survival, Reproduction, and Dispersal
C. Biological Interactions

1. Host range.
2. Interactions with and effects on other organisms in the environment, including effects on competitors, prey, hosts, symbionts, predators, parasites, and pathogens.
3. Pathogenicity, infectivity, toxicity, virulence, or as a carrier (vector) of pathogens.
4. Involvement in biogeochemical or in biological cycling processes (e.g., mineral cycling, cellulose and lignin degradation, nitrogen fixation, pesticide degradation).
5. Frequency with which populations undergo shifts in important ecological characteristics such as those listed above.
6. Likelihood of exchange of genetic information between the modified organism and other organisms in nature.

IV. Proposed Field Trials

A. Pre-Field Trial Considerations

Provide data related to any anticipated effects of the modified microorganism on target and nontarget organisms from microcosm, greenhouse, and growth chamber experiments that simulate trial conditions. The methods of detection and sensitivity of sampling techniques and periodicity of sampling should be indicated. These studies should include, where relevant, assessment of the following items:

1. Survival of the modified organism.
2. Replication of the modified organism.
3. Dissemination of the modified organism by wind, water, soil, mobile organisms, and other means.

B. Conditions of the Trial

Describe the trial involving release of the modified organism into the environment.

1. Numbers of organisms and methods of application.
2. Provide information including diagrams of the experimental location and the immediate surroundings. Describe characteristics of the site that would influence containment or dispersal.
3. If the modified organism has a target organism, provide the following:
   a. Identification and taxonomy.
   b. The anticipated mechanism and result of the interaction between the released microorganism and the target organism.

C. Containment

Indicate containment procedures in the event of accidental release as well as intentional release and procedures for emergency termination of the experiment. Specify access and security measures for the area(s) in which the tests will be performed.

D. Monitoring

Describe monitoring procedures and their limits of detection for survival, dissemination, and nontarget interactions of the modified microorganism. Include periodicity of sampling and the rationale for monitoring procedures. Collect data to compare the modified organisms with the nonmodified microorganism most similar to the modified organism at the time of the trial. Results of monitoring should be submitted to the RAC according to a schedule specified at the time of approval.

V. Risk Analysis

Results of testing in artificial contained environments together with careful consideration of the genetics, biology, and ecology of the nonmodified and the modified organism will enable a reasonable prediction of whether or not significant risk of environmental damage will result from the release of the modified organism in the small-scale field test. In this section, the information requested in sections II, III, and IV should be summarized to present an analysis of possible risks to the environment in the test as it is proposed. The issues addressed might include but not be limited to the following items:

A. The Nature of the Organism

1. The role of the nonmodified organism in the environment of the test site, including any adverse effects on other organisms.
2. Evaluation of whether or not the specific genetic modification (e.g., deletion, insertion, modification of specified DNA sequences) would alter the potential for significant adverse effects.
3. Evaluation of results of tests conducted in contained environments to predict the ecological behavior of the modified organism relative to that of its nonmodified parent.

B. The Nature of the Test

Discuss the following specific features of the experiment that are designed to minimize potential adverse effects of the modified organism:

1. Test site location and area.
2. Introduction protocols.
3. Numbers of organisms and their expected reproductive capacity.
4. Emergency procedures for aborting the experiment.
5. Procedures conducted at the termination of the experiment.

Index

About the Editors and Contributors

THE EDITORS

Joseph Fiksel is a Senior Scientist in the Research and New Product Development Division of Teknowledge, Inc., and is Program Manager for Risk and Decision Systems. Prior to joining Teknowledge, Dr. Fiksel organized and directed the Decision and Risk Management unit at Arthur D. Little, Inc., in Cambridge, Massachusetts. He is a recognized expert in the assessment of technological risks to human health, safety, and the environment. Dr. Fiksel received his M.Sc. and Ph.D. in Operations Research from Stanford University, in California, and his B.Sc. in Electrical Science and Engineering from the Massachusetts Institute of Technology. He also received a Government of France fellowship for advanced research at the University of Paris, and is fluent in the French language. He is an active member of several professional societies, and recently founded the New England Chapter of the Society for Risk Analysis. In addition, he has authored over thirty publications in professional and scholarly journals.

Vincent Covello is currently Program Manager for Risk Assessment and Acting Program Director for the Decision and Management Science Program at the National Science Foundation. He has been with the National Science Foundation for seven years. Prior to coming to NSF, Dr. Covello was a Study Director at the National Academy of Sciences and Professor at Brown University. He received his B.A. with honors and M.A. from Cambridge University in England, and his Ph.D. from Columbia University. After graduating, he served as a Peace Corps Volunteer in Nepal in Community and Agricultural Development. Dr. Covello has been the recipient of several awards, including a Woodrow Wilson Fellowship and an NSF Sustained Superior Performance Award. He has authored or edited fourteen books and numerous articles on various topics related to health, safety, and the environment.

173

THE CONTRIBUTORS

Lawrence W. Barnthouse   Environmental Sciences Division, Oak Ridge National Laboratory, Oak Ridge, TN 37831

John Cairns, Jr.   University Center for Environmental Studies, Virginia Polytechnic Institute and State University, Blacksburg, VA 24061

Alfred Hellman   International Trade Administration, Office of Trade Development, Office of Basic Industries, U.S. Department of Commerce, Washington, DC 20037

Stuart B. Levy   Department of Microbiology, Tufts University School of Medicine, Boston, MA 02111

Gilbert S. Omenn   School of Public Health and Community Medicine, University of Washington, Seattle, WA 98195

Anthony V. Palumbo   Graduate Program in Ecology, University of Tennessee, Knoxville, TN 37996

James R. Pratt   Hancock Biological Station, Department of Biological Sciences, Murray State University, Murray, KY 42071

Gary Sayler   Department of Microbiology and Graduate Program of Ecology, The University of Tennessee, Knoxville, TN 37996

Gary Stacey   Department of Microbiology and Graduate Program of Ecology, The University of Tennessee, Knoxville, TN 37996

Richard G. Wiegert   Department of Zoology, University of Georgia, Athens, GA 30602